# WINNING THE FIGHT

# AGAINST DIABETES

By

CHARLES J. MASISON

Publisher – Tomorrows Health Today
445 South Street
Foxboro, MA 02035

John Platt

Health & Happiness

Charlie

## *Testimonials*

I have been receiving testimonials from around the country, Canada, and Europe, from readers of my messages on diabetes, who have read my book. A few typical ones are included here –

Charlie, just read your book, and I agree with most of it without exception. You have done all of us non-diabetics, and diabetics a true service, by being a laboratory yourself (your own body) and pointing out the ways to lower those "readings" from blood samples, as well as the cause and effect using the "scientific method". A great job Charlie!

I have had open-heart surgery, followed by special 8-week course of exercise, nutrition, and stress management. Again, I agree with most of what you say, but I am surprised that a lot of pasta is listed as "low GI foods". Perhaps you are right, and it is good to know.

In the nutrition class were many diabetics who needed to adjust their eating habits. If I should see them on a repeat visit I will pass the word on your book. Again, a great book.

Doug Dartnell
Bow, NH


I liked your book on diabetes a lot. Since many food supplements you mention in it are not available in Hungary, I do not plan to publish it in Hungarian language. I guess more and more food supplements will appear here, and therefore, after some time, it may become useful to publish your book here. I hope you succeed with your book in the US. I think it is great, indeed.

Laszlo Domjan, MD, PhD
Budapest Hungary

Your book describes the logical application of many studies of basic diabetes research worldwide. Your analyses of how your blood glucose levels respond to many dietary alterations is impressive in its detail, and the book clearly explains how you used your own body to sort out which research was most relevant to reducing your blood glucose.

Your book is an excellent reference for those wishing to take a nutritional approach toward preventing or treating diabetes.

Daniel Masison, Phd
National Institute of Health (NIH)
Bethesda MD


I am glad I caught you in. I need three copies of your book. We are having a family gathering, this weekend, and three of my relatives have diabetes. Can you expedite my getting them? The local bookstore is out of them.

Ralph Penney
Mansfield MA


Hesh gave me a copy of your book, and as the expression goes – the rest is history. I had been getting scores averaging in the high 160s. My glucose level this morning was 109, and that is typical. THANK YOU. A couple of months ago, the good doc said that I had diabetes. I thought that it was genetically because my brother and father were diabetics. I took a look at the Atkins books, but the stores were full of Atkins candy, Atkins chocolate milk, Atkins everything. I felt that the plan was more commercial than beneficial and a fad that would go away. I want to thank you for writing the book, and for going through the trouble to have it published. I will recommend it to our friends, and we hope all the good you are doing keeps spreading. Your personal examples, all the home-style advice and reasoning, your questions and explanations, all hit home. This is a level headed, easy to understand book, that makes sense and not just a fad by some famous doc trying to cash in.

Bob Weiner
Attleboro MA

# WINNING THE FIGHT AGAINST DIABETES

CONTENTS                                                                PAGE

Information is out there, for us to discover
that could change our lives, forever.

Charles Masison

## *A Self Help Program That Works*

This book assumes that you, or a loved one, has diabetes, or wants to avoid getting it. You need help. This is the only book you will need to fight diabetes. This book is different than any you may have read, or heard about, on diabetes, or diets. It is the only book, now known, that tells how an adult diabetic <u>successfully fought the battle</u> to rid himself of diabetes.

The American Medical Community, and perhaps others in the world, in the 1999 time frame, will tell any interested person, that diabetes cannot be cured. They will say the cause of diabetes is a gene, virus, or an accident/injury. This book uncovers the enemy in the current, diabetic epidemic threatening our world, and shows that this enemy can be overcome.

It is the story of how the author actually rid himself of diabetes, without following the traditional medical approach of taking medicine. He also did not follow an exercise program. Most often, when someone is diagnosed with diabetes, they are told to take medicine for the rest of their life, and get deeply involved in any exercise program. In using research from around the world, and in using his body as the test lab, the author developed the successful program described herein. The hope and desire this book represents, is to lead diabetics away from this debilitating disease to non-diabetic, healthy lives.

It is a self-help book in that you cannot achieve the same results without direct participation in the process. It contains explanations and much data.

The tabular data especially, can be taken from the book and posted somewhere convenient to remind and guide you in the program. The reader will live the program, step-by-step.  The book emphasizes the self-healing process that a reader can follow in taking responsibility, on a daily basis, for their own health.

The author presents the first self-test program that works that leads the diabetic to a progressive improvement in their diabetes.

The program was built upon a man's fight to overcome the disease, who had training in the scientific method of analysis, developing experiments to obtain test data, and having the willingness to take risks with his own body to establish credibility of the approaches.

A prestigious American clinic has provided the empirical data that shows the credibility of the program.  Achieving credibility was a sigh of relief, but not surprising, in that the nutritional approach described in this book is based on information from some of the world's leading nutritionists.  Going to those sources was necessary because many of America's doctors did not have the opportunity to take nutrition courses in medical school.  Also, much of the world's useful research on nutrition was being conducted outside the United States.

The Fight Diabetes Program, is built upon  the discovery of what you should, or should not be eating, or drinking, to rid yourself of diabetes.  It also includes certain supplements that are needed in the fight against diabetes.  Because stress plays a role in diabetes, this book provides approaches to stress reduction as well.

There are 18 million Americans diagnosed with diabetes.  There is about a million more joining those ranks each year.  That is 80,000 a month.  It is a true epidemic.  In addition, there are others with diabetes not included in the 18 million.  Those persons are diabetic, and have been attacked by this silent killer for years.  They have not had a glucose test to identify themselves as such.  They may be working next to you, or even members of your family.

These undiscovered diabetics need the described program in this book, to prevent the serious complications of diabetes, amputation, blindness, and kidney failure. The hope is that unknown diabetics will be identified as such, and put on a program to rid themselves of diabetes before this silent killer has too big a start on them.

Our bodies are not waiting to age to get diabetes. Baby boomers in their 40s are being diagnosed as diabetics. This group had a 79% increase this past year. They need the tools to fight diabetes too.

Diabetes has become a major threat to a healthy life throughout the world. In seeking information that could help me, I discovered that in Australia, there are 1.2 million diagnosed with diabetes. I understand that in other countries, the number far exceeds this.

There are many down-to-earth additions to the basic Self Help Program that provide further depth to the book. The books contains useful information for diabetic prevention, and for the juvenile diabetic. It also identified some information for general health that can be helpful in developing and maintaining a healthy body.

It is a book not to be missed if you have diabetes, or know of someone that does. You don't want family and friends joining the diabetic club where the initiation fee is an amputated foot, blindness, washing out a kidney three times a week, or heart disease.

Get started on the fight to rid yourself of diabetes. The Self Help Program is the path to get you there. Why am I so confident in saying this? Because I used this program to take my dangerous glucose reading from a reading of 168, and still climbing, to a consistent 103-108, 12 to 17 points below the safe number of 120. The Self Help Program works!

## *The Fight Begins*

On taking my annual physical, at a well-known, well-respected clinic, I was told by my primary physician "You have tendency to diabetes."

"How do you know?" was my quick response.

"Because your glucose level is 146", said the doctor.

"What's glucose and how did you find my number?"

"Glucose is sugar.  Remember we took some of your blood?  The number is the amount of sugar in your blood."

"OK, but what is the good number, and the bad number?"

"200 and above, is bad, and 120 is good."

"I'm close to good!"

"Here's a prescription for some medicine, and an appointment with a nutritionist!" That ended the conversation, and thus started my hunt to find out what is this enemy called diabetes, and how does one fight it!

It is always a frightening feeling to find out you may have a terrible enemy inside you.  I experienced this sudden realization that I could be in serious trouble.  It wasn't cancer, but it sure didn't sound good, from the look on the face of my doctor.  I immediately felt that if something like this happens to any of us, that we need to learn as much as we can about what it can do to us, and also learn how we can stop it.  I was a fighter and didn't just want to proceed on a treatment plan of medicine.

In looking forward to what I must do to combat diabetes, I intuitively wanted to look backward. What happened for me to get diabetes? How do people "get" cancer, or heart attacks? How is it that some people, lots of them, don't get diabetes, cancer, and other diseases?

Did I do something to get it? Did others do something to get it, and like a cold, I caught it? If I could win out against the current "attack" of diabetes, could I get it again?

I wanted to know!

The first counter attack against the enemy is knowledge. In preparing for a battle, a general, admiral, commander, or chief, has to have knowledge. This includes:

- The understanding of the battleground.

- An assessment of the enemy's strength, and his unique capabilities. This assessment is based on intelligence, which is an information gathering activity.

- An assessment of his resources, as compared to the enemy's strength.

- A strategy, and a plan, to win.

The same is true for the approach to winning the fight against diabetes. I needed to learn, and others must learn, what is happening in our bodies now, and what would continue to happen, and what, if any serious complications would happen in us. That included the prospect of an early death. I needed to understand this disease and what I could expect from the medical community, to assist me in my fight. Are there expert diabetes fighters that I can locate? I wasn't given the knowledge of the cause of my diabetes, by the clinic, just knowledge of a standard treatment plan. That plan was to take a certain medicine for the rest of my life. I didn't see myself as the standard patient. I would become an active participant in my health care. I decided to solicit medical information wherever I could locate it, even from around the world.

Winning the battle against my current attacker will not be enough. I must stop the cause of diabetes.

## *Fighting What?*

Being told that I had diabetes, I knew something was wrong with my body, but I didn't know what. What is diabetes? What damage can it do? How did I get it? Can I get rid of it? If I am in danger, I want to fight it, but I need more information. Let's start with what happens when any of us are told that we have diabetes.

## *The Serious Complications of Diabetes*

I learned that this disease has serious complications. It is a progressive, silent killer. It keeps getting worse! It has reached epidemic proportions. Doesn't anyone know how to stop it? Very few doctors have the answer on how to even lessen its affects. America spends almost as much money on Diabetes, as Cancer, 98 billion to 107 billion.

There are long-term serious complications – The National Institute of Health (NIH) reports that undiagnosed diabetes has caused millions to lose their vision. In addition, complications of diabetes are the third leading cause of death in the United States. Yearly, diabetes in the U.S. causes about 12,000 new cases of blindness, about 4,000 cases of kidney failure, and about 20,000 have a foot or leg removed. Diabetics are 2-4 times more likely to have heart disease, and 60-70% have mild to severe forms of nerve damage. It puts you on a path to severe physical limitations, and death. Wow, that got my interest real quick.

## *The Awareness of the Battle*

I was in a battle. I was sprinting for survival. I could not allow my body to deteriorate with too much sugar circulating in my bloodstream each day. I could not take the, "I will do something when I can get to it", attitude."

Being in a fight, not only for my quality of life, but also for my very life, I came to realize that if I were successful, others would benefit. My family, friends, and others in this world, would also benefit.

They would benefit if they could understand what I was going through, and why, and not be paralyzed by the needed disciplined effort, or the lack of a personal goal to achieve, and participate in the success.

This realization propelled me to seek out every possible source of diabetic information. I would then try various treatment approaches on myself, and then record the experience. It meant taking every daily opportunity to explore, analyze, and record. It sometimes meant developing a hypothesis, a guess at truth, and then finding a way to wrestle it to the ground of reality.

## _Beginning to Understand the Disease_

I discovered that it is known as a silent killer, because it is inside you. There are no broken bones, rashes, bloody noses, etc., to provide visibility, like other health problems. The symptoms are subtle, quiet. You can have it, and not know it. You could even be experiencing some of the symptoms and either not take them seriously, or attribute them to some other health condition.

About 18 million Americans have diabetes. There are many others who do not know they have diabetes. It sort of sneaks up on you. Until recently, I didn't know that I had it. And yes, if your glucose number is over 120, you have it. My glucose readings say I have it. I discovered that diabetes is not like cancer. But both can lead to a painful and shortened life.

There are very large differences, as to suspected causes, and treatment. I began to suspect that if I have diabetes, I must take an active role in my treatment plan.

There is much being written lately about a diabetes epidemic. About 1,000,000 new cases in America are diagnosed each year, and that number appears to be increasing. There is not enough proven research to fundamentally guide you, in preventing, mitigating, or eliminating it. There are many conflicting reports on how to treat it. There is no "magic bullet" or pill to rid yourself of it.

Why is there a diabetes epidemic? Diabetes is not contagious. I learned that it takes years to appear in our bodies, at least measurable. Some consider it a constant presence. I would hope that it can be reduced or eliminated. The only answer must be that we are causing it individually, and because we are all doing it, because of life style, environmentally, etc, we are causing it collectively. That is the epidemic.

In a recent article in <u>Parade Magazine</u> titled "Should you be checked for diabetes," it states that diabetes has increased by 79% among 30 to 39 year olds in recent years. Teens are now developing diabetes, a disease that usually happens to adults over 40.

The fact that diabetes is now occurring in younger adults, not just in seniors, suggests that whatever we are doing, it is not waiting for our bodies to age, in order to occur. It doesn't necessarily need the deficiencies of certain minerals, in aging bodies to manifest itself. What could cause this? Might a major shift in our eating habits, that occurred hundreds of years ago, be the reason?

Could it be that we went from being meat eaters, to eating mostly farm products? We have grown more crops than ever before. Many of these crops are used by manufacturers and processed into foods. We have more snack and "junk foods," more canned goods, more cereals, more bottled drinks (with often much added sugar). We, means Americans, first because of our large food production capability, and then the rest of the world population. However, the Australians have 1.2 million diagnosed with diabetes. There are African countries with many more than this.

While we are questioning, if there are more diabetics in America, is it because the low fat diet, and resulting increase in eating carbohydrates, is a contributing factor?

In any event, it would appear that our epidemic is self-caused, and that we can begin by modifying our eating and drinking to remove ourselves from this major health concern. If this approach works for large numbers of us, it will be like letting the air out of the balloon, and the epidemic will drift away.

## _How is Diabetes Treated Now?_

I rather quickly gained a lot of knowledge, from medical reports (about 12-14 a month), and discussions with diabetic patients, and some doctors. I came to understand that many in the medical community are generally in awe of the disease. Many state that it is mysterious. Their assumption of the cause of diabetes is a gene (you inherit it), a virus, or an injury. The enemy to be fought is not clearly identified. This made it difficult to engage the enemy on the field of battle.

There was a further complication with gaining knowledge from the medical community. The community did not speak with one, consistent voice. Richard Bernstein, M. D. of the New York Diabetes Center, is a well-known, respected voice in many of the pieces of the diabetes puzzle.

Dr. Bernstein takes issue with the American Diabetes Association (ADA). He points out that the association felt that dietary fat caused a rise in cholesterol, which caused diabetes, and therefore a diabetic should reduce fat in their diet, and substitute large amounts of carbohydrates (carbs). Dr. Bernstein said that there never was a study that supported this position.

The doctor further says that even though recent studies support the concept of less carbs, the ADA continues to recommend eating large amounts of carbs, including rapid-action carbs, such as table sugar, bread, potatoes, pasta, and to follow this with very large doses of insulin.

This is one medical expert identifying a medical association advocating the wrong approach, from his research and patient experience. Why, was the ADA apparently wrong? Who knows? Even though the ADA hypothesis sounds incorrect, it must have been based on some database, at one time. The importance of the diabetic fighter is that there is difficulty in establishing a feeling of credibility with sources in the medical community.

## Current Medical Practice

Patients usually discover that they have diabetes by a physical exam given by a doctor. They must have the initiative to schedule an exam on a periodic basis. This is usually a general exam, as most patients do not have awareness that they might have diabetes.

On discovering the diabetic condition, most physicians in America will prescribe medicine. Many will advise the patient to make an appointment with a dietician. This is because most physicians have not had nutrition courses in medical school, because these courses were not part of the regular curriculum. We know this by other doctor's statements now appearing in the print media.

The physician, in informing the patient that they have to take medicine, tends to prescribe a popular medicine, like Glucophage, and directs the patient to take 500 mg every day for the rest of their life. The key point is that after diabetes diagnosis, the doctor usually starts treatment with a standard approach. This approach is usually based on the latest pharmaceutical research that has developed medicines for a treatment plan. Given a lack of any other treatment knowledge, the physicians are preceding on the informational base that they can work with, which at this time is very limited for this disease.

## *Controlling the Diabetes*

I found that the medicines available to most physicians, for most physical ailments, are those that pharmaceutical companies have convinced them are appropriate. For diabetes, the problem is that the prescribed medicine is meant to "control" the disease, i.e. stabilize it to a certain level, rather than to eliminate it. I subscribed to many health publications, browsed the Internet, and everything I read in my basic research stated this.

In watching a national TV show, the actor said, "Medicine is not a cure, it just <u>controls</u> the symptoms." This is an example of the media stating the same thing. What it means to me is that the objective of the medical community is to bring the patient's glucose level down to a "safe" level and reduce the affect of the serious complications discussed earlier. Maybe, but this should not be the goal. The goal is to change a diabetic to a non-diabetic.

The second problem of the medicine approach is the potential side affects. When I opened my package containing the prescribed medicine, there was a paper from the pharmaceutical company. It said a percentage of the people that use the medicine die. No thanks; I did not want to take the risk. There may be some taking it because they are more afraid of the disease, or they have complete reliance on their doctor. This is OK, but the doctor can only do the best he/she can with the limited knowledge he/she has.

A majority of the diabetics I talked with told me that most doctors send the patient to a dietician. I was sent to one. This was just after my primary physician prescribed medicine for me. After 45 minutes of earnest questioning by me, I got up and left, telling the dietician that she did not give me any specific information to help me. I was completely frustrated. I didn't know what role nutrition played in diabetes. For example, I didn't have any new information to fight my battle. I didn't learn what not to eat, what to eat, and how to tell the difference.

In discussions with others on a treatment plan, the treatment usually proceeded to monitor their glucose. I learned that one acquaintance was told to take medicine, take readings when fasting, after meal, and at bedtime. She was testing 5 times a day, 7 days a week. Her fingers looked like pincushions. The other directive from the doctor was "go see an eye doctor."

Treating the results of diabetes, not the cause. Because of a limited knowledge of cause and affect, physicians are left with a program of trying to "control" the diabetes. That word comes up again, and again, in reading the literature. I have not seen any statements from physicians that talk to eliminating diabetes, i.e. getting below a 120-110 glucose reading. If they did, one of those would have written this book!

Also interesting, in discussing diabetes with doctors and patients, I never heard of or from a doctor, who knew exactly what caused diabetes for any patient. I did learn that they all had treatment plans, and the goal was to <u>control</u> one's diabetes, to a certain value. The value seemed to be determined by their evaluation of the current state of the patient, rather than evaluation of the cause of the diabetes for that patient.

The American Diabetes Association has stated that 120 was the standard good glucose reading to shoot for. Several treatment centers say 110, and that seems to be the new preferred standard. How do we know if 120 or 110 is the right number? Where was this proven, and how?

The usual treatment approach is the admonition, check your diet, and get more exercise. OK, <u>what diet</u>, and what <u>exercise</u> program, should be followed? Together with prescribing medicine, this appears to be most doctors' preferred treatment approach.

There are many good doctors, clinics, and hospitals. In my search, I have gained confidence in their ability to treat the patients who are diagnosed with diabetes. What I was looking for in my ability to fight this disease, is not a treatment plan to reduce the problems of the serious complications of diabetes, as they progress to further disability, but how to stop the progression, and reverse it.

### *What we Know About the Enemy*

I reasoned that in order to fight an enemy, we need to know a lot about that enemy. This is difficult with a silent killer! Most of us don't know that we have diabetes until we get an abnormal glucose reading on a physical. I never thought that I had diabetes. I had heard a little about it, but that was it. This enemy has a big head start on me, like occupying large chunks of territory (my body).

As I approached this task, I knew very little as to <u>why</u> some people get diabetes. We do know what could happen in our bodies <u>if</u> we get diabetes. We will suffer through the serious complications of the diabetes and leave this earth early.

We have an idea how our body works, and can somewhat understand this disease that has invaded our body, even if this is not a complete picture, and in some aspects, not a very clear picture. That is okay, as long as it provides a way of attacking the disease.

Let's look at our body processes, and see who gets diabetes, and what are the types of diabetes. And, after understanding how the medical community currently treats diabetes, we most likely will see the need for a self-help program, if we are going to win this battle.

> "We need to question our suppositions
> And subject them to the scientific method"
> Dr. John Clarkson, Dean, Univ of Miami Medical School

## *What Happens in Our Bodies?*

One of the benefits of being a graduate of MIT, is learning to use the "scientific method". This is a disciplined approach to solving what you don't know. Scientists, engineers, and also those in the medical community, practice it. You hypothesize a theorem, postulate, or a guess. You then conduct research, experiments, and then analyze what you find out to see if you gain more insight into the validity of your "guess".

This is the approach I used in trying to understand our body processes. I subscribed to many health publications, rode the Internet, talked to many people, etc. I read biological information on the body, and gradually developed my own way of expressing how diabetes must occur, and some thoughts on what I could do about it.

Our bodies use the food we eat, to make the sugar we need for energy. We eat some food, or beverages, and the digestive process in our body, converts them into sugar. As the sugar enters our bloodstream, our pancreas is alerted and produces insulin. Insulin helps the sugar leave the blood and go into our cells. It acts like an escort in getting the sugar into the cells, where it is used as a kind of fuel. When this happens, the way it should, the level of sugar in the blood goes down, and our cells produce energy for an active, and full life.

When we have diabetes, our bodies cannot always make energy from the food we eat. Sugar stays in the blood instead of going into the cells. Either the pancreas does not secrete enough insulin, or our cells become resistant to insulin. When the blood sugar cannot get into the cells, it leads to very serious complications of diabetes. We don't want to lose a leg, go blind, or have serious heart problems.

The digestive system operates like an assembly line in reverse. Assembly lines usually take many parts and combines them into a product. The digestive system takes whole goods, and using digestive juices, breaks them down into their chemical components. The result is small absorbable nutrients that can be utilized by our cells, so they can generate energy required to maintain life. It usually takes 24 hours, or longer, after a meal, for food to go through the digestive tract.

Figure 1 (next page) shows the flow of food through the digestive tract. The digestion process actually starts in the mouth where saliva does some pre-processing. Because this happens, it suggests we eat slowly giving the saliva a chance to work effectively.

The food continues to the stomach and beyond, into the colon. Each does some of the processing. It is clear to see that this is a complete digestive processing system.

We have an organ called a pancreas. It is about the size of a hand, and lies next to our stomach. When food starts changing to sugar (glucose), an alert goes out to the pancreas to start making a hormone called insulin. The job of insulin is to get the glucose into our cells.

When this process is normal, (Figure 2), the insulin is at the cells to help the cells process the glucose. They help the cells "open its entrances" or turn on "its receptors". The glucose enters and our cells take the glucose and convert it to energy.

If there is a lack of insulin at a cell, the entrance receptors are either not open, or not many of the cells have their receptors open, to take in the glucose from the bloodstream. In order to maintain our need for energy (even the movement of our eyes, tongue, hands, etc), we would need to receive insulin from outside our body, through injections.

Insulin could be there, but none, or only a few, of the receptors could be open. This may be a case of over-saturation of insulin. Because of what we eat, and how we eat, our pancreas may be working too hard to produce lots of insulin. This could overwhelm our cells trying to extract

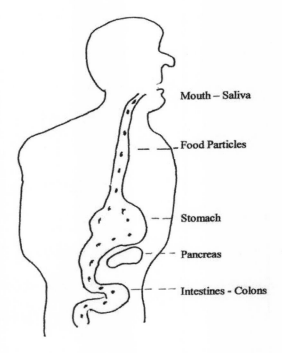

Mouth – Saliva

Food Particles

Stomach

Pancreas

Intestines - Colons

The digestive system

Figure 1

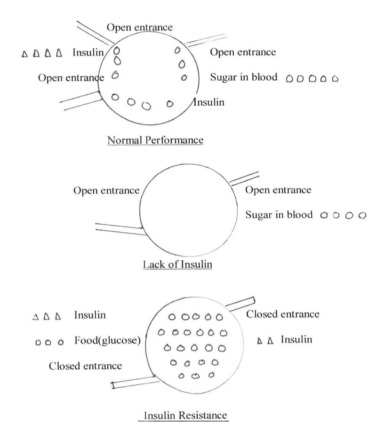

Figure 2

all of our glucose. It develops into insulin resistance, by our cells. It's also possible that our pancreas can slow down like any tired worker on an assembly line, and produce less insulin.

These are three cases of glucose to cell processing. It is a process, and needs to run efficiently, if we are to have a healthy body, and all the parts must to their job, as an integrated whole. Throwing a cheerleader up in the air, and catching her, needs all the performers working correctly, and in unison with each other.

A sure sign that this is not so in the food digestion process is indigestion. This often occurs when eating too much, too fast, or eating the less desirable foods, from a processing point of view. From seeing the figures, and understanding the process, you will understand some of the points I will cover later.

I have described part of the process from the eating of food, or drinking a beverage, the processing happening in the digestive system, and the interaction of insulin and the cells. Now, let's look at what happens in our cells.

Inside the cells there is a furnace. It is called the mitochondria. Each piece of glucose in the cell is burned as fuel by the mitochondria, and produces energy. We need this energy to even wiggle a finger.

You may wonder how a physical thing, the glucose particle, becomes energy. When we put a physical thing, a log of wood in the fireplace, it burns. It produces two kinds of energy, heat and light.

The mitochondria furnace, like any other furnace, needs to be turned on. The thyroid performs this function, when activated by the hypothalamus, a gland that is controlled by the brain.

## _Our Bodies Reaction to Glucose_

I was learning fast. I had to at least develop some understanding on how our bodies worked. In particular, I needed to know how bodies reacted to the output of the digestion system. I then needed to express this knowledge in my own way, and not in complex medical terms.

For the majority, diabetes means having an elevated blood sugar level. I learned that insulin resistance can occur, and that insulin could not clear out all of the excess sugar in our bloodstream. I also came to realize that if my glucose reading was above 120, I was allowing free radicals to exist in my body. These free radicals could produce the serious complications that I was trying to avoid.

My body and subconscious mind was busily trying to help. My body's instinctive reaction was to try to clear all of the excess glucose from my blood. It can do this by stimulating my kidneys to excrete large volumes of urine containing the glucose. This is why thirst, excessive drinking of liquids, and frequent urination are classic symptoms of diabetes. As a result, there is massive excretion not only glucose rich urine, but massive losses of nutrients, including B1, B6, B12, and minerals: magnesium, zinc, and chromium.

Losing these nutrients is perhaps the primary reason for the deterioration of your eyes, kidneys and peripheral nerves, which often occurs with diabetes. Nutritional supplementation of our diet is the key to avoiding, minimizing, and even reversing the diabetes, and its harmful effects.

## *Who Gets Diabetes?*

Anyone and everyone can get diabetes. <u>You</u> can have diabetes. We are all humans, living in similar environments, eating popular foods of this generation, and affected by stress, and lack of exercise.

Millions of Americans have diabetes, and do not know it. This must be because many new cases of diabetes are being discovered each year. Also, the severity of the disease may indicate that a person may have had diabetes for a while.

It has been reported in the well-known Nurse's Health Study, of more than 43,000 women, "those with waist of 36 inches or more, were 5 times more likely to develop diabetes, than those of waists, of 26 inches." It went on to say "abdominal fat appears to be related to insulin resistance, where your cells don't respond to insulin." Apparently this resistance causes your pancreas to stop producing insulin, resulting in diabetes.

In reading this, it seemed to me that the cause-affect is likely to be the opposite of abdominal fat causing diabetes. Based on what I have analyzed so far, my guess is that you develop diabetes, and therefore get abdominal fat.

There doesn't appear to be much merit in causing those who are "chubby" to develop anxieties about their waist. Also, the study doesn't say they eliminated, or included, those who have larger physiques, who naturally have larger than 26 inch waists. Let's take the scientific approach rather than use a correlation technique that can link two variables. We can relate two or more variables by statistics that can prove almost anything, but doesn't really identify the cause-affect relationships.

Your body cannot process enough of the sugar that gets converted from the food you eat, and you get diabetes. An excess of the quantity of food, or the wrong type of food, appears to be the problem. In addition to causing diabetes, it stores fat in your abdomen.

A treatment plan for the condition may not be to reduce fat in fear of getting diabetes, but to use the abdominal spread as an <u>indicator</u> that we have to begin to mitigate, and then eliminate diabetes.

It is interesting to observe that there are now significantly more non-obese diabetics. This may be because there is more testing going on than before, and what is being observed is diabetes in its early stages.

Early on then, I felt that diabetes was not caused by genes, virus, or injury. By saying family members have, or had diabetes, and therefore we are apt to get it, was simply not true. It doesn't make sense. It also takes away all of the blame from us, our eating habits, etc., and puts the blame on outside sources. I began to believe that it was more likely environmental than heredity.

Recently, I heard on the radio that there are people getting ready to sue the major food providers, like the fast food chains, for their getting fat and developing diabetes. Whether this claim has a solid basis or not, it is clear that these people believe their diabetes and obesity are caused by what they eat.

Let's find a way to defeat this disease, by finding the cause, and stopping others from getting it. We also need to slow down the progression of the disease, for those who have it. And lastly, we have to crush this enemy by eliminating the diabetes. Our enemy is not the fast-food outlets, but the lack of information as to the dangers to our health.

## *Types of Diabetes*

Very simply, diabetes is a condition of the body, when there is too much sugar in your bloodstream. There are basically two types of diabetes. The first type is known as type I, juvenile, or insulin dependent diabetes. In this type, the body makes little or no insulin. People with this type must take insulin shots to live. A small percentage of people with diabetes have this type of diabetes. This type occurs most often in youngsters, or adolescents and therefore is called juvenile or insulin-dependent diabetics.

In the second type, the body does make insulin, but cannot use all of the insulin it makes. This seems to happen after the age of 40. Those with this type of diabetes are the larger percentage with diabetes and are often referred to as adult, or non-insulin dependent diabetics.

Generally, the symptoms for either type are the same, and include:

| | |
|---|---|
| Increased thirst | Dry, itchy skin |
| Increased passing of urine | Numbness, tingling in hands, feet |
| Increased hunger | Blurred eyesight |
| Feeling very tired | Sudden weight loss |

I found it interesting to see the symptoms; the increase in thirst, and increase in passing of urine. These are the traditional symptoms of diabetes, going back to the Greeks, who labeled the condition, diabetes, their word for "passing through." The word insulin in Greek is for island. The groups of inslet cells in the pancreas that are responsible for making insulin, and other hormones, look like tiny islands under a microscope.

Let's sum up what we know about the process of food to glucose, and glucose to energy. The following diagram may help.

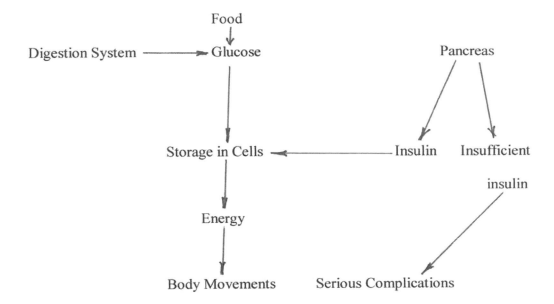

When everything works the way it should, when we consume food, it ends up as potential energy in our cells, so that we can make body movements. This can be a wave of our hand, or running fast. If there is insufficient insulin to do its job, there are immediate serious complications such as fatigue, difficulty in breathing, confusion, coma, and death.

Juvenile diabetics need to have insulin injections to move glucose into their cells. This is their regular, daily, practice. They live this pancreatic condition every day.

About 10% of diabetics are hypoglycemians. This is a person who normally has a small amount of glucose flowing in his/her bloodstream. Their glucose level is normally around 70 milligrams per deciliter (mg/dl) of blood. These persons are in danger of not having enough glucose in their bloodstream. They are below the 70 mg/dl. Common symptoms include feeling dizzy or faint, or unusually nervous or confused. If this happens, they need to add glucose quickly. Knowing that they are hypoglycemians, they may carry candy bars, or glucose tablets to eat quickly. It would also be a good idea to carry their glucose test equipment with them to take a quick reading, when symptoms occur, and 15 or 20 minutes after taking the sweets. If they don't know that they are hypoglycemians, then discussing symptoms with their doctor would help.

In general, the serious concentration of the medical community on hypoglycemians having too little glucose in their bloodstream, has led many doctors away from seeing the serious problem of the hypoglycemian having too much glucose. The reader will learn more on this in Chapter XIV.

The other 90% of diabetics are hypoglycemians. Their glucose levels are normally around 120 mg/dl. There is sufficient glucose to avoid near-term complications. Their potential problem is long-term increases in their glucose level, which can lead to the serious complications of neuropathy, macular degeneration, and kidney and heart failure.

Also interesting is that the lack of sufficient insulin for glucose storage in itself, can cause a reaction in another part of our bodies. The body then looks to our other cells, the fat cells, our long term depositories for future famines, etc. When this happens, a substance known as ketones or ketacids are produced as a by-product of the breakdown of fat in the energy generating process. These ketones will make the body acidic, and cause the same serious problems, that the hyperglycemian person has.

"Nutrition is the Best Medicine"
Hippocrates

### *A Very Important Discovery – Nutritional Healing*

In October 1999, I had my yearly physical. I was told I had a tendency to diabetes. They knew this from the sugar present in my blood. I was told that the bad number was 200 and above, the good 120, and that I was 146. I later came to realize that as long as you were over 120, you had the enemy eating away at your body, from within. I was further told to obtain the medicine glucophage, and to take it daily, for the rest of my life.

I paid for, and proceeded out of the pharmacy with the glucophage. It was a coincidence, in that picking up the medicine, that I saw the book on nutritional healing. It turned out to be one of the best purchases I ever made. It provided me with my first insight into fighting diabetes.

Finding that book was like someone saying to me, you now have a sword, go fight your enemy. At that time, I envisioned my enemy as diabetes, a big read and black dragon. Hey, a shield might come in handy too.

I sensed that this discovery of a nutritional approach was as if the Olympic gods had decided I should get a chance to beat this enemy, diabetes. It was a very big coincidence that I should walk out of the store, carrying the glucophage, exiting by the correct aisle, to just happen to see the book, *"Prescription for Nutritional Healing."*[1]

Someone learning that you have the symptoms of diabetes, and knowing of this book, may provide you with a similar sword to fight your battle. You may later think of this person as your guardian angel. You may also wonder about such things as coincidences.

---

[1] Prescription for Nutritional Healing, Phyllis A. Balch, James Balch

In opening the book, I found that it was like a catalogue, with a listing of applicable supplements for a large number of illnesses and diseases. I was anxious to try the supplement approach and see if it could help me in my fight to rid myself of diabetes.

My glucose reading was now up to 168, and still on an upward trend.

Using the section on diabetes in the booklet, I went to a health store and purchased a small supply of recommended supplements.

I had been taking supplements for a few months, when I saw a quote by the glucophage manufacturer, that reported some serious side affects, including death, for some who had taken the medicine. I had decided never to take the medicine. I am sure that my primary physician was unaware of this caveat by the pharmaceutical. In any case, the medicine was not for me. I would agree that the probability of death may be a relatively small number, and that glucophage helps some people, however I didn't like the possibility of death. I had too much to lose in my life.

I returned to see my physician in about 3-4 months. My doctor was pleased that the medicine had resulted in a reduction of 15 points. I stated that I had not taken the medicine, but had taken the supplements of anti-oxidants, minerals, and vitamins. My primary physician never blinked an eye. She quietly, and professionally, accepted this information. On later visits, she encouraged me to continue whatever I was doing, as it was achieving results. I didn't know it at the time, but this "treatment" was to become one of three cornerstones of a nutritional approach that helps you fight diabetes.

Taking supplements was prompted by finding *"Prescription for Nutritional Healing"* by Phyllis and James Balch, (reading list). To treat diabetes, they emphasized the need to take supplements. I also researched the definition of the supplements. I found research that said some supplements were replacing key nutrients being depleted in our bodies by advancing age, or the need for them was because some people had diabetes.

The Balch's developed their recommendations based on research into patient's responses to various supplements. They were well qualified to do so. As a certified nutritional consultant, from the American Association of Nutritional Consultants, Phyllis has been a leading nutritional consultant for almost two decades. She continues to study nutritionally based therapies, procedures, and treatments developed worldwide.

Dr. James Balch is a graduate of Indiana's School of Medicine. He established a practice as a urological surgeon. He became a fellow in the American College of Surgeons. He is a pioneer in combining traditional surgical treatments with nutritional approaches.

## *If We Got It, We Must Heal With Supplements*

The first battle I saw to be fought with this enemy diabetes, was to defeat the current enemy, the known enemy now in from of me. I am not sure where this enemy gets its foot soldiers, or its weapons. This is the same medically, as saying, I don't know what is causing the problem, but I think I can treat it. In war, soldiers usually have some kind of Field Manual that they use as a guide. My manual in starting to counterattack was the Balch book on nutritional healing.

The Balch's recommended taking supplements for diabetes. They divided the supplements into the three groups of essential, very important, and important. The recommended dosages are for adults.

### Essential –

| | |
|---|---|
| L-Carnitine (empty stomach) | 500 mg twice/day |
| L-Glutamine (empty stomach) | 500 mg twice/day |
| Taurine (empty stomach) | 500 mg twice/day |
| Chromium Picolinate | 4-600 mcg/day |
| Zinc | 50 mg/day |
| Quercetin | 100 mg 3x/day |
| Vitamin B complex | 50 mg 3x/day |
| Biotin | 50 mg/day |
| Inositol | 50 mg/day |

This data from PRESCRIPTION FOR NUTRITIONAL HEALING by James Balch and Phyllis A.Balch, copyright © 1997, 2000 by Phyllis A.Balch . Used by permission of Avery Publishing, an imprint of Penquin group (USA) Inc.

This is where I started with a program of supplements. I had immediate positive results. Some of the daily numbers went up and down, like popcorn in a cooker. However, I was happy to be gradually lowering my number. Later, I added some of the next groupings.

**Very Important –**

| | |
|---|---|
| Coenzyme Q 10 | 80 mg/day |
| Magnesium | 750 mg/day |
| Manganese (w/o calcium) | 5-10 mg/day |

**Important –**

| | |
|---|---|
| Vitamin A | 10-15,000 IU/day |
| Vitamin C | 3-6,000 mg/day |
| Vitamin E | 400-1,200 IU/day |

A subsequent publication, "The Super Antioxidants", by Dr. James Balch (reading list), added:

| **Additional recommendations** | **Daily** |
|---|---|
| Alpha Lipoic Acid | 300-600 mg |
| Potassium | 99 mg |
| Vitamin B 3 niacin | 100 mg |
| Vitamins B 6 | 50-100 mg |
| Vitamin B 12 | 1,000-3,000 mcg |
| Bilberry Grape Seed Extract (200mg) | |
| Garlic and onions | |

I added most of these over a month or so.  I grew to understand the value to my body from taking some of the supplements.  The proof was in the reduction of my glucose levels.  Some will accept the fact that the supplements work, because the author won the fight against diabetes using them.  Some will need to understand how the supplements help fight diabetes.

General examples of how the supplements affect the body are –

A deficiency can help cause diabetes –
Zinc, Glutamine, Magnesium, and Manganese

Aids in the release of insulin –
Taurine, Quercetin

Normalizes blood sugar –
Lipoic acid, C-Q-10

Aids in proper insulin utilization –
Chromium

I have recently seen three other supplements mentioned in several writings.  The one that I have heard the most about is gymnema sylvestre, which is an ayurvedic gurmar item.  This has been very popular in India in treating diabetes and other medical problems.  There is a Chinese bitter-melon called Momordica charantia, and the third is a prickly pear cactus called opuntia spp.  I have added gymnema and feel that it has helped.  I obtained it at a natural-food store.  These three supplements might be available at some mail-order sources.

There is much more detail to follow in the book as to how supplements fight diabetes.  Taking the different supplements gave me an advantage in my fight against diabetes. Think of it as my army of foot soldiers now fighting against the enemy's foot soldiers. It was obvious that I needed as many warriors as the enemy.  Therefore, I took the recommended dosages.  The research behind the Balch's, said that was the amount that needed to be taken, and that's what I took.  Success started to follow.

## _What Vitamins, Herbs, and Trace Minerals Can Do for Us_

If you have diabetes, like I did, taking supplements is a good idea. You need them to avoid the potential serious complications that will probably occur. You don't want to be blind, have kidney failure, etc. Supplements have the capability to mitigate, or even eliminate the disease. There are a number of them to take. I found that the best way to take them was to space them out during the day. Also, it helped to be consistent. Some like taurine, glutamine, and carnitine are best taken when fasting. They appear to do the most good before a meal. I added chromium, alpha lipoic, and the other essential supplements at the same time. Taken the first thing in the morning seemed to work best for me, and this became the anchor for my daily fight against diabetes. C-Q-10, magnesium, manganese and the others were taken together later in the day. Because they need to be taken twice daily, I take the second helping of taurine, glutamine, and carnitine, later, by themselves. I take both the fasting, and the later in the day supplements, with a 16 oz. glass of water. This meets the objective of daily drinking large quantities of water. If concerned about "drowning" the supplements and their losing their effectiveness, you may want to start by drinking a third of the water first, and then start taking the supplements.

There are certain supplements packaged together, by the pharmaceutical companies. These could be any two or three on our list. This sounds good for convenience, but most often, the quantities, in mcg's or mg's are less than recommended, for the diabetic. It wouldn't work for me, or another diabetic. I was taking the amounts to correct a problem, not just maintaining myself in good health. The quantities can be reduced when I bring my body back in control.

As an example of pharmaceutical packaging, I purchased a bottle of 90 tablets of "Doctor's Choice for Diabetics," at a local health store. Wow, this should be great. I could take 14 supplements in one tablet. Carnitine, glutamine, taurine, and inositol from the Balch "essential" list were <u>not</u> included. Going on, C-Q-10 was not listed from the "very important" list, and A from the "important" list. There could still be a gain from the other 8 items. But, chromium was 200, not 4-600 mcg, zinc 7.5 not 50mg, biotin 1 not 50 mg, magnesium 100 not 750 mg, and so on. Not one made the recommended item or amount recommended by Balch.

When we drive an automobile, we are taking the gasoline from its tank and providing it to the engine. When there is no more gasoline, the automobile stops. We cannot take a few supplements now and then. We need a constant flow of good stuff (nutrients, etc.) to fuel our cells (our engine). In taking the supplements, I found that some health stores like GNC, had some of their supplements packaged in different quantities than recommended by the Balch's.

In the list of essentials, chromium picolinate came in 200 and 400 mcgs. I took them together to make 600 mcg. Zinc came in 30 mg. I took one tablet, not 50 mg. I did not take quercetin, vitamin B complex, biotin, or inositol. I felt that I got enough quercetin in the food I eat. I didn't feel comfortable with the vitamin B complex, and I couldn't find biotin or inositol.

In the list of very important, C-Q-10 came in 30 mg, and I took 3 of them for 90 mg. I took 500 mg of magnesium and 10 mg of manganese. This is the size they come in.

In the list of important, I took 10,000 of A, 2,000 of C, and 800 of E. I could only find alpha lipoic in 100 mg units, and I took 4-6 units, usually 2-3 twice a day. I took 99 mg of potassium, 100 mg B6, and an occasional 500 mg B12. I also took bilberry, grape seed, and garlic now and then. I spread taking the supplements throughout the day.

Wow, some of you must be saying, and are you kidding?
The effort to do so, and the cost, must be prohibitive. Maybe an operation to remove a leg, or a funeral is cheaper, but I don't know, and don't anticipate knowing in the foreseeable future. I am convinced that diabetes is nothing to fool around with. You have it, you get rid of it!

## *Herbs and Other Recommendations*

Next on the fight to overcome diabetes, was the discovery of herbs. There are many herbs that contain antioxidants. The most potent have flavonoids, which are found in almost all plants.

One that seemed to make sense for me was bilberry. It is an anthocyanidin-rich herb. It has strong antioxidant effects. Blueberries and purple grapes have similar capabilities. Bilberry is locally grown in New England, and is a cousin in the plant family to blueberry and cranberry. I was later to learn that locally grown food seems to be more advantageous to our diet. This is usually true throughout the world.

Bilberries are very good to counter diabetes. They protect our eyes and circulatory system. Dr. James Balch states, "There is nothing in this pathological high sugar condition that cannot be solved with bilberry. Diabetes causes microcirculation problems all over the body. Bilberry has been shown to be the best hope available to diabetics facing vision impairment. Bilberry has proven effective in healing macular degeneration." Bilberries also contain other important antioxidant minerals, zinc, manganese, and selenium.

I take bilberry as a supplement, and add blueberries to oatmeal, and other foods. I drink cranberry juice. In discovering the importance of flavonoids in our diet, I also discovered the value of grape seed extract and pine bark extract. Some come in the form of pycnogenols. They all can be purchased from General Nutrition Centers (GNC), as well as from health stores, and some drugstores. I added them to my program, and take them from time to time.

The following may be helpful to add to your supplements.

Bilberry    Blueberries    Cedar berries   Huckleberries

Pycnogenol or grape seed extract

Spirulina    Garlic   Kelp

The Balch's suggest that you do not take cysteine. They say, "It has the ability to break down the bonds of insulin and interferes with absorption of insulin by the cells."

The herb fenugreek is well known to the Mediterranean, and throughout the Middle East. The herb there is used as a cure for diabetes. Gymnena is a woody, climbing plant common in central and southern India. Its Hindu name, gur-mar, means "destroyer of sugar." Gymnema is used in traditional Ayurvedic practices. It is manufactured by Nutraceutical Corp in Utah USA. Both of these herbs are excellent additions to the supplements. The suggested dose is a tablet, twice a day, with Taurine, Glutamine, and Carnitine.

## *Trace Minerals at Work*

Why are trace minerals a part of a supplement program? These minerals are not anti-oxidants fighting the oxidized free radicals. Why do we take a group of "iums" including chromium, magnesium, selenium, potassium, along with zinc and manganese? Our source of these minerals is in the earth that our foods are grown in. Medical reports being circulated say that our bodies cannot process zinc from the food we eat. The actual fact may be that the zinc doesn't exist in sufficient quantities anymore in the ground from which our food is grown. These minerals are almost depleted in many of our areas for growing foods, in many parts of our country, and in other countries. There are studies that are reporting analyzing trace minerals that include zinc, potassium, chromium, and calcium, among others. These results show deficiencies of these trace minerals in our food supply that are causing severe loss of protection in our bodies against infection, diabetes, cancer, and other problems we see emerging today.

Many of us are being affected by the loss of minerals in our diet. The baby-boomers are now being diagnosed as diabetic. They had an increase of 79% last year. What does this mean? They are being raised from an early age that has a very poor nutritional program for them. This includes eating food, unknowingly, that are deficient in trace minerals. For example, in Southeastern USA, studies indicate that the inhabitants are now more susceptible to dangerous diseases, because of a lack of certain minerals in the food chain, and in particular zinc and selenium.

It makes sense to me to take mineral supplements to "replace" the lack of them in our foods. The program that I developed that led me to being a non-diabetic, was built on using information from nutritional experts from around the world and analyzing those inputs that worked effectively. It was a try-it and see, self-help approach.

We have identified what supplements to take in our fight against diabetes, and what they do in helping us win this fight. They worked for me in creating a movement of my glucose reading to a safer level.

Medical research is on going. I try to stay tuned to it. Some of it results in insignificant changes, some fairly small adjustments. You will find in the appendix the results of some supplement small modifications. They are the result of adapting new information into our program, and verifying positive results. It continues the focused path of discovery. There is a Modified Supplement List in the Appendix.

I have passed on to you, the reader, the basic information in describing the three building blocks of the supplement program, as part of your new approach to create the fighters you will need to fight the enemy. We will now take a look at <u>why</u> you should take them, and where identified, at what dosage.

## *Why We Should Take These Supplements*

If anyone is already taking prescribed medications for diabetes, and would like to take some of the supplements I take, you should let your physician know. He may want to determine if there should be an adjustment in your medication. He might also want to use a "try it and see it" approach, adding supplements to your program. If successful in his practice, he might wish to help spread the word on the benefits of supplements for those who may be edging towards diabetes, but not there yet.

My reasons that supplements are important to me are:

- My glucose # went up to 168 before I got started with supplements, and I needed these fighters to halt the increase.
- Once I started, they were quick to slow down, and halt, the upward progression.
- When my body is deficient in some, like manganese, it can be at least a partial contributor to an increase in my glucose level.
- Some supplements, like taurine, help release insulin to carry blood sugar to my cells, or like chromium, help in the utilization of insulin by my cells.

I think the reasoning to take supplements goes beyond these four reasons. I call it the "fighter theory." I asked myself, what are anti-oxidants that Balch discusses, really all about. As long as I am above the "normal" glucose level, then something is happening in my body that is not normal. I am being attacked! I am in danger every day of being attacked, and my body is heading toward problems with my heart, kidneys, eyes, limbs, etc. Wow, it is that simple.

I understood very easily that diabetes could cause the external problems of neuropathy (leading to loss of limbs) and macular degeneration (leading to loss of sight). But how does it affect the kidney, and is it serious? All the blood in my body passes through my kidneys. There it is. My bloodstream has to pass through some kind of a processor. This processor has thousands of filters removing wastes and excess water from my blood, and they become part of the urine I pass.

Lots of sugar in the blood causes my kidneys to work harder. This will eventually cause some filters to degenerate and the wastes will start to accumulate in the body. It's like having the garbage pile up in your house when the trash company is on strike. I would then have to take dialysis treatments, or have a kidney transplant. With dialysis, you might be able to control the problem. Once a kidney is damaged, it can't be repaired, but may be replaced. To avoid this, I understood that I must control my sugar. A periodic urine test is probably a good idea too. In addition to the process of damaging a kidney, I learned that when my tissues are exposed to high glucose levels they will, sooner or later, be attacked by the enemy. There is a process in which free radicals (the enemy) are formed. Free radicals can damage cells, nerves, and blood vessels. This leads to the danger to my limbs, eyes and heart.

Okay, let's see if we can produce some of our fighters to minimize oxidation. We need to bring antioxidants into our bodies to counterattack the free radicals. Many herbs contain antioxidants. They have potent little fighters called flavonoids, and are found in almost all plants. Bilberry is one example. Bilberry also contains the antioxidants, manganese, zinc, and selenium. Other little warriors are pycnogenols, such as grape seed extract. Vitamins C and E are also antioxidants. There are others. Perhaps the most important for me is alpha lipoic acid (ALA). It is a very powerful antioxidant. Also, like wounded soldiers coming back to a home base, C and E can have their antioxidant properties restored by ALA. The list of antioxidants goes on, C-Q-10, blueberries, garlic, etc. I wanted these warriors working for me. That's the fourth reason I take supplements.

When we have diabetes by eating too much, or too much of the wrong food or beverages, we will have excess glucose in our bloodstream from our digestive system, and our pancreas will have difficulty in performing in an optimum way.

The excess glucose in our bloodstream will oxidize, requiring anti-oxidants to fight off the formation of free radicals. If our glucose reading is above the safe level, we will need fighters. Supplements provide these fighters.

Our self-healing program is based on reducing the input of bad stuff, and using supplements when we don't stick to the approach or unknowingly take something that is not good for us, i.e. lemonade.

Before we go further, we have to have a clear understanding whether we are discussing ridding yourself of diabetes as an interesting theory, or a practical plan of self-healing. If from an intellectual theory, point of view, stop reading and give this book to someone who can use it.

You can't just leave the information in this book. It has to be put to use to help you fight this disease, before it overcomes you. Make a copy of significant data, such as the list of supplements you should take. Tape them to the inside of your medicine cabinet door, or wherever you are, when you take the vitamins, herbs, and minerals.

You are following a self-help approach and you should look for ways to customize the approach to make it your way of best meeting your needs in achieving optimum health.

## _Supplements in Action_

In my hunt for ways to defeat diabetes, I gathered much information on what supplements do for us. I didn't have to rely on faith that they were essential, very important, or important. We look at what supplements do and see how they can specifically help us in our battle against diabetes. The supplements serve us in several ways, including helping in insulin production and utilization.

<u>Taurine</u> – aids in the release of insulin. Diabetes increases the body's requirements for taurine. Taurine works with zinc in maintaining eye health. A deficiency may impair vision. <u>It is vital for the proper utilization of sodium, potassium, calcium, and magnesium.</u> Also, it helps to prevent the development of dangerous cardiac arrhythmias. Works exceptionally well in helping to lower high cholesterol and high blood pressure.

<u>L-Glutamine</u> – especially taken with C and E, is a potent detoxifier at the cellular level. Glutamine levels fall with advancing age, and this has been linked with a wide range of disease, including diabetes, and heart disorder. Can enhance mental functioning. Decreases sugar cravings, and desire for alcohol. Do not take if you have cirrhosis of the liver or kidney, or Reye's syndrome.

<u>L-Carnitine</u> – reduces the health risks posed by poor fat metabolism associated with diabetes. Prevents fatty buildup, especially in the heart, liver, and skeletal muscles. Enhances the effectiveness of vitamins C and E. Men need more carnitine than women.

<u>Chromium</u> – The average American diet is deficient in chromium. The ability to maintain normal blood sugar levels is jeopardized by the lack of chromium in our soil and water supply, and by a diet high in refined white flour, sugar, and junk foods. Chromium picolinate has been used successfully to control blood cholesterol and blood glucose levels.

This essential mineral maintains stable blood sugar levels through proper insulin utilization, important for people with diabetes.

Chromium is vital in the body's utilization of carbohydrates, protein, and fats. Fat is turned into extra energy for us. This also helps in losing weight. Many vitamin manufacturers package chromium and vitamin C together. <u>You should not take them together.</u> It won't hurt you, but vitamin C interferes with the absorption of chromium. The chromium simply passes through your system without benefiting you. You will wonder why the supplements are not helping you more than the readings you are getting.

<u>Potassium</u> – This mineral is important for a healthy nervous system, and a regular heart rhythm. It also regulates the transfer of nutrients through cell membranes. This transfer capability decreases with age, which may account for some of the circulatory damage, lethargy, and weakness experienced by older people. Signs of potassium deficiency include insatiable thirst, fluctuations in heartbeat, glucose intolerance, high cholesterol, and insomnia. <u>Tobacco and caffeine reduce potassium absorption.</u>

<u>Magnesium</u> – Assists in calcium and potassium uptake. With B 6, helps to reduce and dissolve kidney stones. Deficiencies can result in insomnia, rapid heartbeat, and poor digestion. A magnesium deficiency can be synonymous with diabetes. The consumption of alcohol, the use of diuretics, the presence of fluoride, high levels of vitamin D, all increase the body's need for magnesium.

<u>Zinc</u> – Zinc levels tend to fall off as we age, and therefore zinc is related to various problems associated with aging. The decline in zinc levels in our bodies is said to parallel the decline in the immune system, and that corresponds with aging. I believe that the reason it corresponds is because seniors have been eating foods longer that are deprived of zinc in their soils.

Zinc plays a vital role in the production of insulin, and therefore adding this supplement to our diet is essential.

Also, once the disease is underway, zinc can relieve some of the complications of diabetes, especially vision loss. This is important to know, and to use zinc while you are moving from a diabetic, to a non-diabetic. Sufficient intake and absorption of zinc is needed to maintain the proper concentration of vitamin E in the blood. A deficiency may result in fatigue, hair loss, high cholesterol, memory impairment, and a propensity to diabetes. Do not take zinc and iron supplements at the same time. Do not take more than 50 milligrams of zinc daily. I take 30 mg.

Vitamin B-12 – It helps in the utilization of iron. It is required for proper digestion, absorption of foods, the synthesis of protein, and the metabolism of carbohydrates and fats. It prevents nerve damage. It assists memory and learning. Strict vegetarians should use B-12 supplements as this vitamin is found in meats. There is some concern in the medical community that cutting back, or eliminating red meat can lead to a B-12 deficiency. This deficiency is associated with spinal cord damage, peripheral neuropathy, and dementia. B-12 dementia has been reported as exactly what you see in early Alzheimer's. B-12 is vital for memory, and brain function. It's a vitamin everyone over 50 should take. However, when B-12 is combined with almost any other vitamin, it becomes destroyed during the digestive process (Bottom Line Health). Therefore take B-12 alone, or only with folic acid. Wait an hour before taking any other vitamins.

In a recent issue of The American Journal of Clinical Nutrition, researchers at Saarland University Hospital in Hamburg Germany found that most vegans, (no animal products), and a majority of vegetarians (ate eggs & dairy), had very low amounts of B-12 in their bodies. Their research showed that 67% of the vegans had abnormally high homocysteine levels, 38% of the vegetarians, and only 16% of the meat eaters. Homocysteine can be a major threat to our hearts.

B-6 – is necessary for the absorption of fats and protein. It reinforces vitamin E. It promotes red blood formation. It is also needed for normal brain function. It aids in the absorption of B-12. A deficiency may result in hearing loss, numbness, dizziness, and fatigue. It is available in some food, but not in supplement quantities.

Manganese – is needed for blood sugar regulation, healthy nerves, and protein and fat metabolism. It is required for normal bone growth. It is needed for the best utilization of vitamins B-1, and E. A deficiency may lead to eye and hearing problems, high cholesterol levels, rapid pulse, and pancreas damage.

Vitamin C – The diabetic with a shortage of insulin, is likely to have cells deficient in vitamin C. A deficiency may also lead to vascular problems for diabetics. Vitamin C may slow or prevent complications that occur in diabetes. Because the body cannot manufacture vitamin C, it must be obtained through the diet or through supplements. Most of the vitamin C obtained in the diet is lost in the urine. When vitamin C is taken with E or A, it makes them more effective in helping your body.

Vitamin E – This vitamin is an anti-oxidant, important in the prevention of cardiovascular disease. It has been said that the higher the level of E in your blood, the less likely we will die of heart disease. This means 800 to 1200 IU's daily, or 2 to 3,400 IU capsules. It improves circulation, and is necessary for tissue repair. Vitamin C helps boost the effect of Vitamin E. Vitamin E has been shown to protect against approximately eighty diseases. Vitamin E affects the amount of warfarin being used to thin out the blood.

Alpha Lipoic Acid (ALA) – may be the ideal anti-aging antioxidant. ALA is an essential factor in the production of energy. It helps protect every body component from oxidative stress. It is good for the diabetic. It normalizes the blood sugar. It protects against glycation, which causes many of the disorders of diabetics. It reduces retinal disease, cataract formation, and peripheral nerve and heart damage. ALA enhances the effectiveness of Vitamins C & E. Because it is both water and far soluble, it can go anywhere in our body.

Co-Q-10 – Your body starts reducing the production of Co-Q-10 when you are about 20 years old. Co-Q-10 helps stabilize blood sugar. Similar to vitamins A and E, Co-Q-10 acts like an antioxidant. It has a crucial role in the generation of cellular energy, is a significant immunology stimulant, increases circulation, has anti-aging effects, and is beneficial for the cardiovascular system. Helps in hypertension, angina, and heart rhythm disturbances.

Quercetin – promotes insulin secretion and is a potent flavonoid that is found in onions, cayenne, grape seeds, bilberry, pepper, garlic, and green tea. Our diets should include as much of these foods as practical. It is also available in the form of a supplement. As a potent antioxidant, quercetin inhibits the production of free radicals (oxidants).

Inositol – This is a vitamin that is recommended by Dr. James Balch and Phyllis Balch. It is one of our warriors to fight the negative affects of having too much sugar in our bloodstream. It helps in the metabolism of fat and cholesterol. It also helps remove fats from the liver. It is also advocated to be excellent for stimulating hair growth.

There is a "hidden benefit" in taking some of the supplements. Some combinations of supplements provide additional value, above each supplement's value.

For example, recent research shows that when alpha lipoic and L-Carnitine are both taken, this is a benefit beyond fighting diabetes. Together, they can help in providing more energy for our bodies, and enhancing our memories. The February issue of *The Proceedings of the*

*National Academy of Science* reported that Dr. Bruce Ames, at Berkeley, is heading up the research.

The two supplements, taken together, improve the cells inner system, which converts the glucose into energy. They enhance an enzyme that generates the energy.

The result of taking the two supplements together, appears to help overcome diabetes, enhance memory, gives an energy boost, and apparently slows down the aging process. If this fact were verified by the continuing research, it would be like discovering the fountain of youth. For the present, I accept the energy boost, and enhancing the memory benefit.

Before going on to explain the specific phenomena of oxidation, I would like to summarize, why supplements.

I benefited, in my fight against diabetes, by taking supplements. For you, these supplements are specifically identified, at the correct dosage, and for three of them, when they should be taken. Many are vitamins, some are herbs, and others are minerals.

It is possible to achieve some of these same results, with foods that provide the same benefits. It is unlikely that you will eat enough of the right foods, and in a consistent day-to-day basis, to win the battle against diabetes.

I researched many medical journals to determine why some of these provide a benefit, and have identified the reasoning for these supplements, and have shared this reasoning with you, so that you would have the confidence in the supplement program.

I was at this point, and now you are, on the right path to winning the battle.

## How does Glucose become an Enemy in Our Bodies?

Cholesterol and glucose create a similar problem in our bloodstream. They don't become dangerous until they oxidize, which can occur over time. Once oxidized, cholesterol becomes solid and can lodge in your arteries, cutting off the blood going to your heart and brain.

A similar process goes on with excess glucose. Excess glucose occurs when the cells are full and don't accept any more glucose, or when the body's insulin has not caught up with the glucose in the bloodstream to escort the glucose to cells that do have the capacity to take the glucose.

Oxidation is the process by which a substance combines with oxygen and then changes to another form. It is similar to the rusting of metal. The oxidized glucose develops free radicals, which are the enemies who create the serious complications of diabetes. The free radicals are the attackers that can damage cells, nerves, and our blood vessels. They can "chew up our tissues." Our extremities are vulnerable, and nerves can be destroyed in your feet and legs, leading to very poor circulation. This is known as neuropathy.

When your blood flows through the tiny veins and arteries of your eye, oxidized particles create physical pressure against the walls of the tiny veins and arteries. This leads to the condition known as macular degeneration and blindness. Specific supplements fight the oxidized particles. For example, Vitamin E is known as a fighter to protect our eyesight.

To minimize oxidation, we take antioxidant supplements. These antioxidants can remove free radicals from our body, before damage occurs. If damage has happened, they can come in to protect, or lessen the problem. Sometimes they give up an electron to a free radical that has one missing, and is causing damage to your cells. Other times, the antioxidant neutralizes the free radical, by combining with it to form a stable compound.

If you have enough antioxidants, the good guys, you win, and you stay healthy.

## *Developing a Total Program*

Once I understood that diabetes was a progressive disease that could lead to very serious health problems and eventually to early death. I knew that I had to find some way to avoid this.

There was never a thought that I wouldn't be successful. It became a goal to stop progressing towards having a serious threat, to a goal of progressing, step-by-step to mitigating or eliminating the threat. I realized that this meant that I had to change. Something was going on in my life that had caused diabetes. You don't catch it from another person.

One choice was to take medicine and treatments. Cancer patients do. Some get cured, some don't. Norman Cousins used humor to help him overcome his disease. This may seem strange, but there is a well-known book (Reading List) that describes Cousins fight against cancer. Also, there is a report in *"Diabetes Care"*[2] of a Japanese study that found blood sugar levels were lower in people who laughed after a meal. They say daily laughter can help control diabetes blood sugar.

It seemed that those who got cured, took an active role in getting themselves cured, had faith that they would be cured, and followed a program that they could believe in.

I learned that diabetes just doesn't happen overnight. It is the progressive result of doing it to yourself. In order to change, I had to figure out what I was doing wrong, or not doing right. The first test was to determine what in my lifestyle could be causing, or contributing to the presence of diabetes. I was on the hunt. I wanted to come face-to-face with my enemy.

I read everything I could find on diabetes. I talked the fight. People who had the disease were not very helpful, as they all just took the medicine and relied on it to "control" the disease. What a terrible word, control, and if you were not under control, you were at fault. I also found

---

[2] As Reported by *USA Weekend, Oct 10-12, 2003*

many health publications, especially from the pharmaceutical companies, also advocating that approach. I had the Lahey Clinic prescription filled at the pharmacy. As I was leaving, I discovered among other books and manuals, a reference book on nutritional healing. You might say I was led to it because of my inner determination to fight the disease.

That book opened the door to the right approach to rid myself of diabetes. The book recommended taking supplements. As I began taking them, I soon recognized that I was at least stopping the upward progression of my glucose level. I was in the high 120's. I wasn't where I wanted to be yet. The number was not low enough, and when it was, it was not too consistent. But I was winning the fight! I could taste the fruits of victory. I had to push the number down more. I never lost the desire, or feeling of accomplishing the end goal, of sliding under that mystical 120.

I needed a complete program to lower my sugar level below the diabetic level, but I would start with the supplements.

As helpful as supplements were expected to be, I intuitively knew that they alone would not be sufficient. They were something you did after the fact, once you were in the fight against diabetes. What I needed was to attack the cause of diabetes. I decided to look at diets.

## *What Diet Makes Sense?*

In my reconnoitering into the vast verbiage that is flooding us with diets, at the very least, from the Mediterranean to Miami, I decided that I had to make up my mind as to what is important to me, and selectively choose what to review and analyze. Very simply, I was looking for the answer that I never got from the nutritionist. It was what food should I eat, and what food should I not eat. It struck me that it was later to be cool to tell a waiter/waitress that my nutritionist doesn't want me to eat a particular item, rather than go into the logic behind my selections.

I found the answer to my question of what to eat, and what not to eat. It is an approach that was largely found with the Australian nutritional researchers. It identified what foods cause a higher glucose reading after eating them. The approach appealed to me because in a review of biology, I had determined that the pancreas was the key. The first step was to determine when the pancreas started to produce insulin during the digestive process, and the second step, was to determine how hard ye little ole pump had to work in processing a particular food. I gave the name, <u>Slow Digestion Diet</u> to the first step, and <u>Reduced Carbo Diet</u> to the second step.

I was thrilled to be on the hunt and beginning to discover a significant cause of diabetes. Supplements could provide fighters to attack the free radicals, which were the product of ingesting the wrong stuff. They could be somewhat successful in this battle but now the objective of eliminating the enemy at its source was coming into focus.

## Slow Digestion Diet

In my hunt for information that could help me, I discovered a rating system that helps determine which foods were best for people with diabetes. The rating system is simply a ranking of foods based on their immediate effect on blood sugar levels.

It is key to understanding this, to realize that different foods are not equal in the effect that they can have on our body's food processing system. This in turn means that they are not equal in their ability to increase the probability of causing diabetes. A small apple will have a safe rating of 38 compared to a small, plain bagel with a non-safe high rating of 72.

The key is the rate of digestion!

Carbohydrates that break down quickly during the digestion process have the highest rated (bad) values. Carbohydrates, which break down slowest, rated (good ) values.

This seemed to make sense when considered against the food processing system in our bodies. Slower digestion would mean less infusion of glucose into our bloodstream, at a given point in time. This allows the pancreas to take on a reasonable distribution load in providing insulin to keep up with the addition of the glucose into our bloodstream. That's my rationale of why different foods create a different response in our digestion system.

I felt that the best source of information on this rating system is the glycemic index (GI), found in *"The Glucose Revolution"* in the reading list. For most people, most of the time, foods with a low GI value, have advantage over those with high GI values. This again is because insulin from your pancreas has difficulty in keeping up with the rate of input of glucose from the high GI foods. How do we know if the GI value of a food is accurate?

I learned that the GI value of hundreds of different food items had been tested on groups of people using a standardized test method, in several testing laboratories around the world.

A group of Australians developed the data for *"The Glucose Revolution."*[3]   I was fortunate to be alerted from another publication, that they existed.  It was the first discover  that a large amount of significant nutritional research was going on outside of the United States.   The Australians built upon some of the work led by Dr. David Jenkins, a professor of nutrition at the University of Toronto, in Canada.

[3] The Glucose Revolution , © 1996, 1998, 1999, by Dr. Jennie Brand Miller, Faye Foster-Powell, Dr Stephen Colagiuri, Dr. Thomas M.S. Wolever, Appears by permission of  Marlowe & Co, a div of Avalon Publishing Group

## The Bad Foods (High GI ) 72-115

| In General - | Glycemic Index |
|---|---|
| Rice and Rice Products | 82-89 (except brown) |
| Potatoes & Potato Products | 75-101 (except sweet) |
| Breads | 76-95 (except pumpernickel) |
| Corn & Corn Items | 75-84 |

| Breakfast Cereals - | 74-89 |
|---|---|
| Some examples - | |
| Corn Chex | 83 |
| Rice Chex | 89 |
| Corn Flakes | 84 |
| Crispix | 87 |
| Grape Nut Flakes | 80 |
| Cocoa Krispies | 77 |
| Shredded Wheat | 83 |

Baked Goods –

| Pretzels | 83 |
|---|---|
| Bagels | 72 |
| Donut w/Sugar | 76 |
| Vanilla Wafers | 77 |
| Graham Crackers | 74 |

Other –

| Parsnip | 97 |
|---|---|
| Rutabaga | 72 |
| Pumpkin | 75 |

| Dates, Dried | 103 |
|---|---|
| Jelly Beans | 80 |
| Tapioca Pudding | 81 |
| Tofu, Frozen, Dessert | 115 |
| Gatorade | 78 |
| Waffles | 76 |

## The Good Foods (Low GI ) 14-55

|  |  | GI Values |  | GI Values |
|---|---|---|---|---|
| **Fruits -** | 25-55 | | | |
| | Apples | 29 | Pear | 38 |
| | Apricots, dried | 31 | Plum | 39 |
| | Oranges | 44 | Grapes | 46 |
| | Cherries | 22 | Grapefruit | 25 |
| | Peach | 42 | Banana | 55 |
| **Pasta -** | 32-50 | | | |
| | Ravioli | 39 | Spaghetti, whole wheat | 37 |
| | Linguini, thick | 46 | Spiral | 43 |
| | Fettuccini | 32 | Vermicelli | 35 |
| | Tortellini | 50 | Macaroni | 45 |
| **Goodies -** | 14-55 | | | |
| | Chocolate Bar | 49 | Twix Cookie Bar | 44 |
| | Popcorn, Light | 55 | Snickers | 41 |
| | Peanuts | 14 | Ice Cream, Vanilla | 50 |
| | Soy Milk | 31 | Chocolate Milk | 34 |
| | Sponge Cake | 46 | Oatmeal Cookie | 55 |
| **Other –** | | | | |
| | Oatmeal | 49 | Yogurt | 14 |
| | Chickpeas | 42 | Yogurt – Fruit Flavored | 33 |
| | Peas | 48 | Carrots | 49 |
| | Barley | 25 | Tomato Soup | 38 |
| | AJ | 40 | Orange Juice | 46 |
| | Lentils | 26-30 | Split Pea, Yellow | 32 |
| | Sweet Potato, boiled | 54 | | |
| **Beans – generally** | 18-32 | | | |
| | Pinto | 39 | | |

## The Not So Bad, Not So Good Foods (Medium GI ) 56-70

| Bakery Goods – | 59-70 | | |
|---|---|---|---|
| Blueberry Muffin | 59 | Oat Bran Muffin | 60 |
| Croissant | 67 | Hamburg Bun | 61 |
| Pita Bread | 57 | Taco Shells | 68 |

| Other – | | | |
|---|---|---|---|
| Raisins | 64 | Pineapple | 66 |
| Pizza | 60 | Beets | 64 |
| Coca-Cola | 63 | Fanta | 68 |
| Macaroni & Cheese | 64 | Cantaloupe | 65 |
| Couscous | 65 | Honey | 58 |
| Green pea soup | 66 | | |

In my hunt for nutritional information, I looked outside the United States. I found Australians who were worldwide leaders in analyzing and in developing a rating system called the glycemic index. This was an important, additional piece of intelligence in our fight to rid ourselves of diabetes.

Their empirical testing provided rating for over 700 foods that many people in the world eat. The lists above are a compilation of high, low, and intermediate GI items, that I developed from their data, to give the reader an idea of the digestion rate of some popular foods. You can use these, add, or subtract from these, or make-up your own lists, from their book, *"The Glucose Revolution"*. You can obtain a copy from Amazon, if not available in a local library. Check out watermelon. You are in for a surprise.

Take the lists you will use and put them on your refrigerator, or wherever there is a handy spot where you prepare meals. You can use the GI to customize your meals, retaining the "good" foods you usually eat, and avoiding the "bad" foods. There may be recipes in print that you can use, just check them against the GI, and your desires for what you, and your family likes to eat.

I feel the goal is not to eliminate all carbohydrates, but to be selective in choosing which, to eat. I also learned, by trial and error, that you do not have to eat every meal with only low GI items. It became logical to try having a meal that was balanced with a combination of high and low GI foods to achieve an intermediate GI, from time to time. That seemed to work.

The authors of *"The Glucose Revolution"* state that the American Diabetes Association (ADA) supports the emphasis on the quantity of carbohydrates in the diet. However, "The ADA has not recognized that differences in blood sugar responses among foods – the Glycemic Index of foods – are large enough to warrant any change to the current system of carbohydrate counting." In using the scientific method and using my own body as a test laboratory, the results that I achieved support the authors of *"The Glucose Revolution."* I will describe the test results of using the G.I. index later.

To understand ADA's position, I realized that they are basically a clearinghouse for information. They cannot commit resources to basic research. They take data from many sources, and evaluate what they believe is the best recommended approach to date. They must continually assess new information, such as this book, and amend previous recommendations if this book is helpful to the diabetic.

In looking at another source of expertise, Andrew Weil, MD, the best selling author of *"Spontaneous Healing"* and *"8 weeks to Optimum Health"* (reading list), praises *"The Glucose Revolution."* He states, "Here, at last, is a book that explains what we know about the glycemic index and its importance in designing a diet for optimum health." Should we follow the GI as a guide? We are our own test laboratory. I decided to try the guide and see the results.

As a starter, I decided to eliminate, or reduce the amount of white bread, white potatoes, white rice, and corn. Several health studies that I had read reinforced this decision. These four items appear on the High GI Food list with GI's of 76-95, 75-101, 82-89, and 75-84 respectively.

This is at least about 30-60 GI points too high.  There went the mashed potatoes and gravy.  I realize that this will come as a shock to many people, as it did me.  However, in using the glycemic approach, I had early success and went on to implement this technique.

I gradually learned that not all wheat bread is really wheat bread.  In reading labels, I discovered that some breads labeled wheat, were actually white flour with additives.

I had a conversation with a lady who was a fairly recent arrival in America.  She was raised in Albania.  In discussing food, she told me that her Albanian doctor was against his patients eating any pasta.  Pastas are made from different ingredients.  Those in the "good" list have been tested as good.  Just looking at their GI numbers will tell you two things.  One, their numbers are within the good range of 14-55.  Second, the pasta numbers are not all the same, which suggests that they are made of different ingredients.

Using the Glycemic Index helped me decrease my glucose number another 10-12 points.  I was winning the battle!  I was in the 110-113 range, most of the time, but strangely, not always.

Using the supplements and the Glycemic Index was getting me excited to see what else could be used to help me in my battle.  My goal was still in front of me.  My target was to be in the 103-105 range, consistently.

## _Rationale for the Slow Digestion Diet_

The physician's recommended diabetic diet has traditionally been to exclude sugar. Perhaps this was because diabetes usually is associated with too much sugar in the blood. This theory has proven to be wrong. Fifty grams of carbohydrate eaten as white potatoes, causes a higher rise in blood sugar than 50 grams of sugar.

Fatty/protein foods do not increase your blood sugar levels. Only carbohydrates (carbs) do this. In recognizing that various foods have a different impact on our body's processing system, we know that we need some rating system to classify the impacts, if we are to defend ourselves from eating the wrong foods. We finally come to the answer to the question that I asked of the nutritionist. What foods should we eat, and what foods should we not eat.

In Australia, Jennie Brand-Miller, and her colleagues authored the most definitive, comprehensive, and authoritative data source that rates over 700 foods. This rating system, known as the glycemic index, is described in _"The Glucose Revolution"_ (reading list). This glycemic index is adding more food items each year. The research on a food's GI rating is now cooperatively supported by research labs in America.

It may be of interest to know the credentials of the authors of _"The Glucose Revolution"_, Jennie Brand-Miller, PHD, is an associate Professor of Human Nutrition at the University of Sydney in Australia. Thomas M.S. Wolever, M.D., PHD is a professor of Nutritional Sciences University of Toronto, Stephen Colagiuri, M.D. is head of the Department of Endocrinology, Metabolism, and Diabetes at the Prince of Wales Hospital in Australia, and Kaye Foster-Powell M.N. & D. is also an accredited Nutritionist-Dietician in Australia.

I accepted their rating system, as my guide, and have been very successful in using it to reduce glucose in my blood stream. I first started following the G.I. system in early 1999 and first wrote about it that year in my book, _"Rid Yourself of Diabetes."_ I understand that other authors have now discovered this index, and some use it to develop recipes. I think that in general, that is a good idea. If you start by comparing what you like to eat now, against its rating in the glycemic index, this will tell you which items are OK, and which you should avoid, or eat/drink in moderation. You may not have to convert your meals and drinks to some formulated recipe. For some though, it may open new avenues for combining healthy foods into an interesting recipe.

I came to believe that the way to healthy eating is to eat foods that only require my body to process these foods slowly. This gives the pancreas pump opportunity to put out insulin in the quantity, and in the same time interval, as needed, to match up with the digested food, glucose.

The interesting observation is that the G.I. foods matched up with the slow digestion approach .

This book relates my story in ridding myself of diabetes. It is meant for Americans, and everyone around the world that has adult onset diabetes. It is obvious then, that not every population, on every continent, will be able to add a pond of fresh asparagus to a recipe, or cod steaks, and some of the other items I have heard about. The recipe approach has merit though, if it can be used in addition to your regular diet that meets the G.I. approach.

I didn't take the entire glycemic index on faith in my battle against diabetes. I continued my research to find out why an item either enjoyed a good rating, or a poor one. Let's pick a few items, and see if we can identify what it is about some foods that would justify a high GI rating, or an unexpected low rating. This should give us confidence that the GI rating makes sense, and that we should use it in our fight against diabetes.

## *White Rice, Potatoes, Bread*

In using the glycemic index as a guide, the program I followed included not eating white rice, white potatoes, and white bread. Avoiding these foods helped me to become a non-diabetic.

I wondered why. Let's see if we can make sense out of this approach. White rice was not grown as white rice, but brown rice. Evidently when it came across the Pacific ocean, from Asia, then across the continent by rail or truck, it's outer layer, we call the bran, became somewhat rancid. The bran contained the nutrients, vitamins, and also protected the inner white rice. It made commercial sense by the supplier to try removing the outer layer. Evidently milling worked, so that was the way the supplier then shipped it.

Milling is somewhat like peeling an apple. Removing the outer layer, the "bran", resulted in removing the nutrients. The remainder, white rice, when eaten, did not require the digestive system to do much to process it. This then allowed our digestive system to quickly put the "white rice" into our bloodstream. This fast digestion process does not allow the pancreas to input the insulin into our bloodstream in a timely way. Our bloodstream can be compared to a stream of water. As youngsters, we may have put paper "sailboats" in the stream. The boats that came after the first boats, never caught up because the stream kept moving ahead. This is the same with the glucose, converted from white rice, staying ahead of the insulin, and converting to free radicals to attack our bodies.

That's my rationale for not eating white rice. It makes sense to me.

White potatoes appeared to be a similar fast digestion example. Most often, we eat white potatoes without the skins. If we look at mashed potatoes, we see the same problem as white rice. The outer layer, the skin is removed, the potatoes are cooked, and then mashed up. With no skin, there are no nutrients needing processing by our digestion system, and there is the resulting glucose insulin problem. If we look at "fries" or potato chips, we see no skin, and a cut up potato. This is the same problem, and one compounded by the fat, used in the cooking, and fries then dipped in ketchup, which traditionally, contained significant amounts of sugar.

If we bake potatoes and just open them, and just eat what is inside, it appears to be the same problem. If we also eat the skin, it makes sense to me to assume that it is okay, as we are not processing a fast digestion item.

Sweet potatoes are considered okay, and it must be their pulp contains nutrients that need processing. This can be understood when we realize that sweet potatoes are not really potatoes. They are part of a different plant group. Growing in the ground, and looking like a potato, it is easy to understand how they were thought to be a potato. Perhaps the fast food chains will forego their current fries and go to sliced sweet potato fries, fried in fewer fats.

I, at first, left white bread alone in my pursuit of understanding, assuming that the GI must be right, and don't eat it. But, I was curious if it had some rationale like white rice and white potatoes. The dictionary has the answer! It said, "Flour – a soft, fine powdery substance obtained by grinding the meal of a grain, especially wheat, to make into flour." There it was again! Starting with a natural product, and grinding or milling it into another product. I quickly reached the conclusion that the GI was right and to avoid white bread and white flour products.

Still curious, I looked up the definition of wheat germ. It is the vitamin-rich embryo of the wheat kernel that is separated before milling. The more I dug, the more I reinforced the fighting diabetes approach.

## *Vanilla Ice Cream*

For your, and mine, first thought, it would seem that vanilla ice cream cannot be a low GI food. However, it deserves its rating of only 50. It has been researched, as have all of the other food items, by trying it on volunteers who ate it, and then were tested for glucose.

Also, a comparison was made of eating 50 grams of white rice, and 50 grams of vanilla ice cream. The ice cream scored less, a little less than two-thirds of the high score of the white rice.

In further analysis, it was found that fat in the ice cream, essentially surrounded the sugar in the ice cream, and allowed the body's digestive system to process it without injecting much sugar into the bloodstream.

*"The Glucose Revolution"* is a good reference text, and each of us can use the data to customize our diet and develop meals and specific recipes that work the best for us.

## *Reduced Carbo Diet*

The next step I took to help me reduce my glucose level, led to a wide range of health-related scientific reading. I remembered that someone I know was following the Dr. Atkins diet as a program for weight reduction. I was curious and read up on his approach, to see if it had applicability for diabetes.

Dr. Atkins, author of *"New Diet Revolution"*[4], believes that the low fat diet is the underlying cause of diabetes, arthritis, cancer, heart failure, high cholesterol, and the list goes on. An extraordinary statement, and from a cardiologist! Let's look at it logically.

In the 90's, the American medical profession recommended the low fat diet. However, when you reduce fat, you often reduce protein that contains fat. You therefore eat more carbohydrates to obtain all the calories you need. This increase in carbohydrates saturates your bloodstream. Your insulin can't keep up with trying to get it into your cells. This saturation is a large overload on the pancreas trying to pump more insulin to counteract the saturation. This may cause the pancreas to "shut down", or at least go into a state of reduced output, like a tired engine.

Dr. Atkins believes that there is an inability of insulin to do its natural function, caused by too many carbohydrates in the diet, and this results in diabetes, and the other major illnesses.

It is an interesting theory because I know doctors who have said to patients, "you have all of the symptoms of advanced diabetes, including neuropathy, and macular degeneration, but you do not have diabetes." The answer may be that we are all different, and process threats to our

---

[4] New Diet Revolution, Dr. Atkins, Avon Books, 1992

immune system differently. It also could be some other health condition masking or contradicting the diabetes.

Dr. Atkins recommends eating more protein, and less carbs. This protein includes meat, eggs, butter, and other items not allowed in the low-fat diets. The Atkins diet seems to be a dichotomy to me. It has been popular throughout the country, and many claim great success in reducing their weight. On the other hand, there are those in the medical profession who claim his diet is nutritionally unsound, and potentially dangerous. Their analysis seems to start with a premise that Dr. Atkins wants people to start by eliminating carbohydrates altogether, and then keep them cut way down permanently. These doctors feel that eliminating carbohydrates and replacing them with protein and fat can only encourage heart disease, cancer, and a host of other ailments. I didn't arrive at this same conclusion as the critics, but did include references in the reading list for both points of view.

Let's go back to the body's processing of food, starting with the term "insulin resistance." I have heard this term many times, but never a clear explanation. It is too easy to say there is resistance to the insulin, portraying some chemical or other resistance factor. The antidote for this condition is that very often the doctor prescribes more insulin (shots) to overcome the resistance. This may be the solution offered to the non-insulin diabetic who now has resistance, or to the insulin dependent diabetic to increase their dosage. I don't agree with the assumption that the solution is to add more insulin, for the adult diabetic. This reasoning is based on how the body works. The better possibility would appear to be that the cells are saturated with glucose input. They can't take any more! The cells are intelligent. They can simply shut their "doors", receptors. The glucose remains in the bloodstream.

The key is to get the "doors" open. Normally, in order for the glucose to enter the "doors", it needs the insulin to "grab" it and "shove" it through the door. This won't work in this case. The answer might be that the cells must use up some of the glucose inside them by converting it to energy. This means that a need for the energy must appear. The answer, for this condition, must be exercise. Those who have been told that they have insulin resistance should get with an exercise program.

Now let's see if no action is taken for the condition of carb overload, partially or saturated. This is where I believe Dr. Atkins' approach may apply. With an overloaded glucose bloodstream, the body tries to respond. If the cells can't take any more glucose, the glucose goes to the liver's open doors.

The liver forms glycogen from the glucose. When the liver's cells are full, its "doors" close, and the glucose then goes to the fat cells. They are the long-term depositories for protection of the body in times of famine, etc. The fat cells gobble up the glucose and expand. This latest thinking supports my original thinking on the "nurses" study.

As the process of glucose trying to find a "home" continues, the fat cells may have enough, and close some of their "doors". Blood sugar rises, and the body needs water to flush out the system. This then is the thirst and urine symptom of diabetes. With elevated blood sugar for long periods of time, free radicals roam the body and begin to destroy portions of it, creating the serious complications stated previously, and maybe creating the total list of diseases mentioned by Dr. Atkins. Therefore, there may be some validity to his assertions.

My scientific curiosity led me to try a modified version of the Atkins diet. I reduced the amount of carbs in my diet, and ate substantially more eggs and cheese, and other protein than before. This included a fair amount of salmon (influence of Dr. Weil), and other fish, with some chicken and turkey. After six months, reducing carbs and adding some additional protein to my diet, I had a checkup at the clinic and found my heart factors had not changed appreciably. I intend to follow this with another physical in another six months. Probably, the key is not to set out to eat substantially more protein, or as some advise, to arbitrarily balance our plates with one half protein and one half carbohydrates, but to eat only small amounts of carbohydrates to begin with, and add to the rest of our meal needs with protein. I do follow the slow digestion and reduced crab diets as a means of stopping the enemy at its source. We have found the enemy, and it is us! It is not a gene, virus, or the result of an injury. It is what we eat!

If your glucose number is at the non-diabetic level, you may want to take the recommended supplements, as a preventive program. We will discuss the correct dosage later in this book. If in the <u>Fighting Diabetes</u> program, take the recommended supplements. Also, modify what you put in your mouth, for either prevention of diabetes, or to fight diabetes.

It is the combination of supplements, diets, and other factors that I believe has lead to the success that I have had.

## *The Myth of the Low Fat Diet*

Somewhere, somehow, Americans got off the trolley track, when its medical community came out very strongly advocating we go to a low fat diet. The acceptance of this directive resulted in our giving up a lot of our protein. That left us hungry and we reacted by eating more carbohydrates. This helped enormously to fuel the diabetic epidemic.

We are beginning to hear that the famous triangle of what categories of food we should eat, in increasing amounts, is about to be inverted.

We can't let the pendulum swing so far back, that it goes to a dominant protein diet, at least yet. There are some new researchers and authors, who see this movement as the time to promote the theory of the hunter-gatherers versus the produce farmers.

If we can reduce our current practice of eating many carbohydrates, and very little protein, we will impact the whole food chain. The food chain begins with the land in which we grow our carbs. Experts are saying, that in American, we are over producing on smaller plots of land. We are using large amounts of chemical fertilizers and pesticides. Also, that these chemicals pollute the environment and cause erosion by weakening of the soil structure. We evidently are not restoring the land between harvests. A shift to more protein in the diet may provide the impetus for better land management.

The result of all of this is basically simple. We need healthy protein in our diet. There is room for it, as we cut down on those carbs that are not part of a healthy diet.

There are still "experts" believing in the myth, and recommending a low fat diet. This should change as they learn more about nutrition, and how the body really works.

## *Some Thoughts on Food*

There is a surge by many medical practitioners that have name recognition, to become peddlers of various products. Many have their own special recipes for diabetes, weight loss, healthy hearts, etc. This must bring them substantial revenue.

I do not have that interest, as mine is to only bring the word to as many diabetics as possible, that the "silent killer" can be beaten.

I would like to mention a few things about the food we eat that I have learned in the battle to overcome diabetes. We should try to utilize the glycemic index as a guide. Post it on your refrigerator door and refer to it when you can. I want to emphasis that I am not a supporter of the no carbohydrate diet. Our bodies need the fuel they provide to make the energy that we need. It is the correct carbohydrates that are important, as determined by the research that went into the glycemic index, and the research that is still on going.

In the mornings, I like to eat eggs (preferably as omelets or scrambled), cooked oatmeal, or dry cereals. I do not have any form of potatoes with the eggs, and I have a single piece of pumpernickel, or dark rye. As a by product, the omelet without the potatoes, I seem to get more eggs this way, as the cook feels obligated to cover the plate.

I like to get a bowl of oatmeal, mostly made with water, instead of milk. I get another bowl with uncooked blueberries and walnuts. They not only add to the taste, but blueberries are anti-oxidants, and the walnuts are a good source of omega 3's. The waitress now orders "Those Special Bowls". I believe you will like them, and they are very good for you. In addition, oatmeal is good for the heart. There are several good dry cereals. Read the labels closely, and many supermarkets now have separate sections for health-conscious shoppers. Also, organic dry cereals are now on the shelves.

For lunch, I look for tea, natural juice, or water. I will get some salad, an entrée with protein and carbs, and I stay away from flour products, such as sandwiches, and no dessert. I tried eating sandwiches, with the smallest amount of bread. I would buy a Big Mac for example, and discard either the top or bottom bun. Not easy to juggle and eat. I have discovered wraps. Very often they are made of edible vegetable items. The green ones are made from spinach. It's amazing, the wraps usually contain more than a regular sandwich.

For dinners I eat fish several times a week, some fowl and beef, veggies, and salads. I eat some pasta and meatballs, sirloin tips, pot roast, chicken, and haddock, scrod, sole, Alaskan salmon, a fair amount of fish. I have salads and tea or wine. I do not have bread or rolls. I try to have the entrée a la dente – a little cooked.

I also eat a large variety of beans, berries, nuts, some fruit, some soups, but not canned. I avoid cola/soft drinks. It is often difficult, but like Oprah, I try not to eat after 7:30 at night.

We are slowly, and somewhat unknowingly, being enticed into eating larger size fast food or snacks. The fast food companies are apparently trying to attract more customers by offering larger sizes than their competitors.

Many "snacks" are now twice their size of about ten years ago. Family Circle reports –

| Food | Size Then | Size Now |
|------|-----------|----------|
| French Fries | 2 oz. | 4 oz. |
| Bag of chips | ½ to 1 oz. | 2 or 4 oz. |
| Deli Bagel | 2 oz. | 4 to 7 oz. |
| Muffin | 2 oz. | 6 to 8 oz. |
| Soda | 6 ½ oz. | 12 to 20 oz. |
| Candy Bar | 1 ½ oz. | 2 to 4 oz. |

We, and our children, are eating more snack food, as the serving sizes increase. No wonder the American people are increasing in size too.

This may be part of the obesity problem as our population becomes less active, and more like "couch potatoes". We are not working off the extra food amount that exceeds our energy needs.

This can be part of the problem in other industrialized countries too.

"The big concern isn't how much fat, but what type."
Dr. Walter Willett, Chairman, Dept of Nutrition, Harvard Univ.

## *Fat, Good or Bad?*

Fat has been established as the enemy.  We have to be careful what we shoot at, as there are many varieties of fat, not necessarily all bad.

There are two major types, unsaturated, and saturated.  Let's start this rather complicated subject with the "un" fats.  Mono-uns and poly-uns are the good fats.  Monounsaturated fats, are found in olive, canola, and peanut oils, nuts and avocados.  Monos help lower cholesterol.  These fats are not the targets.

Polyunsaturated fats, known as omega 6 and omega 3 fats are known as essential fatty acids EFA's that our bodies need.  Omega 6 is found in sunflower and cottonseed oils, which are used in many foods.  Stores now sell sunflower seeds, which can be eaten as seeds, or you can sprinkle them on other food.

Omega 3 can be obtained from fish.  The fish most recommended are salmon, sardines, mackerel, lake trout, and tuna.  Interesting in that omega 3 can also be obtained in flaxseeds, and walnuts.  Our bodies do not make the 3's and the 6's.  It needs to get them from our diet.  They are important in creating our healthy cell membranes.  These membranes control what enters our cells.  OK, that's the good fats, unsaturated.

The two omegas should be in balance.  With the American diet, and other diets in the world, we get much more omega 6 than we need.  We need to reduce the 6's and increase the 3's.  We cannot just solve the diabetes threat, and ignore the threats to our health system, that hinders the absorption of some of our supplements, and endangers our immune system.  Interesting in that we can't focus on just one part of our body in fighting diabetes.

Fats to be avoided are saturated fats. They are the ones that focused the low-fat diet, without due concern for a lack of protein, which led to the increase in eating carbs. They are believed to raise cholesterol, and cause heart problems. Look out for them in fatty meats, and whole milk products. Milk now comes in skim milk, 1% and 2% fat. Cheeses are beginning to also come in reduced fat content.

A major concern, even more so than saturated fats, are trans fats. We can see the fat on meats when we eat, and we can ask for lean, and purchase reduced fat milk products.

Not visible are the trans fats. Unfortunately, one of the good fats, has been captured by the enemy, and converted to its army. Omega fats/oils have been hydrogenated. This new form is a trans fat and dangerous to our health. Its presence in foods is very common. Read the label on cookies, crackers, and other foods. The labels will often say something like partially hydrogenated vegetable shortening, soybean, cottonseed, and canola oils. Sounds non-threatening doesn't it?

Partially hydrogenated fats start out as polyunsaturated oils, which are then hardened into solid fats like margarine and shortening when hydrogen is "bubbled" into them. The end result is a stable fat with a long shelf life. This is great for manufacturers, not good for us. Researchers estimate they are now in 75% of the foods consumed in the standard American diet.

They are among the enemy we must defend ourselves against. Read labels. Don't eat products that have been partially hydrogenated. They are associated with increased free radical damage. Enough said for me, and I hope for you.

Dr. Walter Willett, Chairman, Department of Nutrition, Harvard School of Public Health, at Harvard University, is one of several who are raising the alarm against products with partially hydrogenated contents. This is one of the many study reports that Dr. Willett's group has issued as a warning to our health.

You still need the good fats, without them, you do not absorb vitamins A, D, E, and K. All of these vitamins you take as food or supplements are not helping you as much as you think they are, when you eat the wrong fats.

## *Overall Viewpoint on Food*

There are certain truths that appear to be self-evident in understanding diabetes. They follow from the questions we can ask.

Do Americans have diabetes because they eat more carbohydrates than protein?

Do we have diabetes because the carbohydrates we eat are not the slow-digestion ones?

Do we have diabetes because much of our food is processed, and not natural?

Do we have diabetes because we overcook the nutrients out of food ?

Do we have diabetes because our soft drinks have large quantities of sugar?

Do we have diabetes because we like to eat large meals, over a long period of time?

Do we have diabetes because we didn't appreciate drinking substantial glasses of water?

Do we have diabetes because new types of food have been created, such as French fries? that is made up of fast digestion foods?

Do we have diabetes because many of our snack foods are unhealthy?

Do we have diabetes because large amounts of sugar are in products like ketchup?

Do we have diabetes because we didn't know that bran is milled away from grain in many of the manufactured foods, leaving a less nutritious food?

Do we have diabetes because we didn't know the benefit of chewing?

Do we have diabetes because we didn't know the benefits of vitamins, herbs, minerals?

Do we have diabetes because there weren't any warning symptoms?

Do we have diabetes because we were put on the path to diabetes as children?

Does America have a larger number of diabetics than Europeans, or Asians, because groceries are not purchased fresh daily, which has led to supermarkets with "processed" products, that contains ingredients to prolong their shelf life, that are not very good for our health?

Many of the 18 million diabetic Americans, would like to take up the fight, if they but knew where to begin.

There must be huge amounts of a particular pain
in the world, that no one seems to mention – the
pain of someone who didn't do their best for a young
person, and can never make it up."

Nuala O'Faolain


## *Let's All Fight For The Children*

As I fought this tough battle of diet discipline, along with the discipline of taking the supplements, I became more aware of the world I live in. I watched others, and began to be curious as to what they ate, and maybe why. I am very sensitive to children, and I began to focus attention on their eating habits.

A recent television ad had a young child advocating two breakfast cereals. One of the cereals is predominately made from white rice, the other from corn. If we <u>do feel</u> that white rice and corn are unhealthy for adults, then we should be consistent, and be concerned of the potential serious complications of diabetes for children. There may be medical reasons why this may not hold true for children, but I do not know of any. We should at least start with developing an awareness with what our children are eating, and concern on the possible diabetic affect on them. We then can look to understand the latest research data to provide answers.

Basically, if we, as adults, don't want to eat certain foods because it will lead to poor health, or serious illnesses, such as diabetes, we should not feed this food to children.

When we desire certain behavior from a child, why do we give them a cookie, a "pop", candy, or ice cream? All have large amounts of sugar. Why do we let them eat pancakes or French toast, and usually with syrup? These foods are made with white flour. Why do we feed them hot dogs, with many believing they are filled with undesirable items, and on a white bun, with sugar-loaded ketchup? Why do we give children, right up to high school age, colas and sodas with large quantities of sugar?  Why do we feed our children potato chips or French fries made of white potatoes?  Why do we feed our children sugar coated (frosty etc.) breakfast cereal?

Are we too lazy, in too much of a hurry to do what is right by our children?  When will we understand that nutritionally poor food can hurt the children, as well as ourselves?

Is it because all of the above food and drinks are easy to store, easy to serve, and strongly advertised?

Think about it.

Recently, I was in a home where a babysitter was looking after a child that was three years old.  This child led the babysitter over to a drawer in the kitchen, and said she wanted a granola bar.  I didn't know what it was.  Bright blue metal-looking wrapper.  I was given one.  It tasted good and I wondered what it was made of.  I checked the ingredients on the wrapper.  The listed ingredients started with white rice, sugar, salt, and high fructose syrup.  The ingredient listing always shows the largest quantities first.  The next ingredients were marshmallow, which was made up of corn syrup, sugar, and gelatin.  Next was fructose, and partially hydrogenated soybean oil.

The mother observed this, and said nothing.  She might as well make the appointment with a diabetes specialist!  Later, I suggested to the mother to throw the big bag full of colorful granola bars away, and on understanding the danger, she agreed.  If pays to read the labels, not only for ourselves, but also for what we feed children.

Another time, I was in a house, and I picked up a wrapper on the floor that had been discarded by a young child.  Instead of just throwing it in the trash, my curiosity got the better of me.  On the outside of the wrapper, that had contained about ten chewy candies, was a picture of those delightful TV characters, Sponge Bob and Patrick.  The list of contents had corn syrup, sugar, and fruit juices from concentrate, modified cornstarch, hydrogenated coconut oil, and carnauba wax. Maybe it's the wax that makes them chewy.

I wonder if the creators of Sponge Bob and Patrick know that they are helping to promote a food item that is very bad for the very children that they hope to entertain?

Many raising children will provide macaroni and cheese, and peanut butter sandwiches. Macaroni and cheese is listed in the not so bad list, and peanuts in the good list. Sounds ok, but lets look at peanuts when they change to peanut butter.

I picked up a jar of peanut butter and read the list of ingredients. It started with corn syrup, sugar and soy protein, and molasses. Lot's of sugar. It then listed 220 mg of salt, and the <u>fully</u> hydrogenated vegetable oils.

The ingredient list suggests we look for better jars of peanut butter, or start writing to the manufacturers. What we normally put on the sandwiches, and what the sandwich is made of, may only compound the problem. And I liked peanut butter sandwiches!

Many of the schools in America, and probably in other countries as well, have vending machines that contain various colas that students can purchase, to go with their lunches. These colas, for the most part, contain large amounts of sugar. In various new accounts, it is reported that schools are reluctant to have them removed. They make a goodly amount of money on them.

Amazing, school administrators, and teachers, stand by and watch money being made at the risk of hurting the health of the unsuspecting children, or their parents. They would gain more respect, if they went to the superintendent, director, or school committee/board, and agreed collectively, to give up a portion of their salary, to meet whatever "need" the school system has for the vending-machine money.

If this does not happen, parents should insist on a deeper scrutiny of the school budget to assess the real needs of the schools. Parents will have to evaluate the alternative beverages for the students. Some students bring juice boxes, the small cardboard box with the hole for a straw, to go with lunch or a snack. These beverages usually have 40 grams or more of sugar. Not the "go to" item. In addition to various bottled waters, coming soon to the market, is water with small amounts of fruit juices, without added sugars.

A mother of a 13-year-old daughter, and a 9-year-old son told me she was not allowing her children to purchase the school colas, nor would she give them the juice boxes. She gives them various bottled waters. She also is waiting on the new product, the water with a small amount of fruit juice, without sugar, or sugar substitute added.

There is a question, in the medical community, of whether diet is a major contributing factor to children's aggressive, and sometimes, hostile behavior. Will the children, in other ways, have to pay for poor nutrition with infections and future diseases? Remember you are usually already sick before a doctor discovers that you are sick.

Each, and every one of us has to join this fight. The children are defenseless. You may not realize the need to help children. You should understand now how to help yourself in this fight against diabetes. You need to change what you feed your kids, and there is a need to spread the word at work, social, or athletic events. If we get to the point where everyone we know is focusing on what is good for our children, it will be like a rock thrown into the pond, with waves spreading out in all directions. It will win the fight for healthy kids!

We may need the voices of those on TV, radio, and etc. with a big enough following to make a significant difference, but let each of us make a start in fighting this fight.

We should also understand that the government could be an ally in this fight, not a contributor to the danger to our children. The government could ban those television ads that are aimed at selling sweet cereal, sugar laded soft drinks, and certain toy-filled-fast-food box lunches.

It may be a stretch to wonder if feeding a lot of the wrong food to a child could be the answer to some juvenile diabetics, but there is some logic that could support this. If a child's pancreas is not fully developed, and is overworked for 10 to 20 months, or more, is it unreasonable to think that it could malfunction and stop producing insulin?

Let's take a look at obesity. It's a major problem in America. It affects not only adults, but our children are more overweight than ever before. Is it a coincidence that diabetes is called an epidemic; at just the time obesity is called an epidemic? The Federal Center for Disease Control and Prevention is saying that poor diet and lack of exercise is now linked with some 40,000 premature deaths. Weight related deaths have increased 33% in the last 10 years. When we win the fight against diabetes, we may be taking a big chunk out of the other enemy, obesity. We save ourselves, and our children.

Each of us must answer the following questions –

Why let the children eat what we have come to understand is not good for us?

Why do we give a child a bad food "goodie" to obtain a change in behavior?

Why don't we recognize hydrogenated items in the majority of food enticing to children?

Why do we not tell others who can feed our children, what our beliefs and standards are?

Let's all fight for the children, ours, and others.

## *The Hero Emerges (Who Me?)*

I have learned a lot about this enemy, diabetes, and how to attack it at its source, and how to gain help once I had diabetes, by taking supplements.

I quickly came to the conclusion that I was responsible for my own health. That means that we are each responsible for our own health. We each have to avoid diabetes' ability to inflict serious harm on us, like the need for an amputation, and blindness.

In reading about American doctors' comments on diabetes, and asking some directly, it came as a shock to learn that they do not know what causes diabetes. They say genes, virus, or injury.

The doctors had two strikes against them. Most were not expert in nutrition. Remember, my primary physician, a doctor at one of the most prestigious clinics in the world, sent me to a nutritionist. Second, it would be very difficult for doctors to generate significant amounts of patient health-data to accurately measure each patient's health.

I began to feel that I had to develop my own self-health program, and that would include a self-examination, self-help approach.

It is amazing! I began to see who the enemy was that was destroying my body. It was me! I also began to see who the hero would be to counterattack this enemy. Again, it had to be me!

I needed a test laboratory to determine what makes the glucose in my bloodstream go up or down. Again, amazing, that the test laboratory had to be my own body. My mind was needed to set up and follow a program of recording and analyzing. No one was going to do that for me.

I would be my own hero!

## *The Self-Test Program*

I quickly developed a theory that diabetes is different. Me, you, we all have to manage our own program. My goal was to rid myself of diabetes, not control it.

I needed to monitor my progress in reducing my sugar level in my blood. In order to do that, I needed to go after short-term cause and affect relationships. If my sugar went up or down, I had to figure out why. Seeing a doctor every several months wouldn't do.

We need the Self-Test Program. It consists of –

- The finger prick technique
- Testing once a day
- Test after fasting
- Record your daily glucose readings
- When readings change from day-day, analyze why, by reviewing food and beverages consumed, and dealing with stress.

I needed a way of measuring if I was successful in various diet and supplements approaches that I was trying on my body. The procedure was to test myself in my home. I decided to do this daily. I found a self-help test kit in the local pharmacy. I needed to obtain a drop of blood, put it on a test strip, and insert the strip in a glucose, hand-held meter. This would give me my glucose number. The usual procedure is to get the blood from your finger. Blood from a cut while shaving doesn't count.

I found that most people, who were self-testing, were using an injector, that contained a small lancet (like a needle) to obtain the drop of blood. You can purchase the injector, lancets, strips, and meter at a drug store, like I did, or at some large grocery stores. Some HMO's will provide a prescription that will save you the cost. Back to the process that I was to become very familiar with. When I was ready to obtain the drop of blood, I inserted a strip in the meter, and then used the injector. I then "scraped" the small drop of blood onto the strip, and read the number. It's that simple.

The procedure is called the finger prick technique. Directions come with the package. You continue to obtain strips and lancets as you use them up. In trying to help others find out if they are diabetic, I let them use my meter, but they use a separate strip and lancet.

I don't have a problem with the finger prick testing. I use the fingers on one hand one week; skip the weekends, and then the other hand the next week. I tell my little finger, you are Monday, and then the others Tues, Wed, Thurs, and the thumb, Fri. Each finger contributes a drop of blood, once every other week.

When you first start out you may need more information to determine what is causing your number. You might wish to test more often. I decided on taking a reading once a day. Daily reading and recordings, should allow me to determine my progress towards bringing my diabetes under control. It was like being in the armed forces where you measured your battlefield success on a periodic basis, and made adjustments when needed.

## *When to Test*

The American Diabetes Association recommendation is generally understood for your glucose reading to not be higher than 120 mg/dl. This is a reading normally associated with "fasting". Therefore, it makes sense to have the test the first thing on rising. For those working midnight shifts, etc, interpret it as before the first meal. The recommended before bedtime reading should be less than 140. This considers the impact of the food you consume during your day. You can also test one to two hours after a meal to see how high your glucose is after eating certain meals.

I didn't follow this procedure because, I didn't want a second, or a third set of finger pricks each day. Also, I recorded a day's worth of food, drinks, and possible stress, the factors that could influence my reading. Then on seeing the next day's reading, I could interpret changes from the previous day's recording as to the <u>cause</u> of any changes. By the way, it was interesting to learn the high sugar content of many of the currently popular bottled drinks.

A high reading is not the only concern. If my reading were below 70, my glucose level would be too low. Glucose is needed by our cells to convert it into energy. Those with low readings could start feeling fatigue, or faint, or go into a coma. If they understand what is happening to them, they would eat a candy bar, or take a beverage that has sugar.

There are two definitions of the person you are, depending upon the amount of sugar normally in your blood. A person who would have a normal glucose reading of 120 is known as a hyperglycemic person. A person with a normal glucose reading of 70, the candy bar person, is called a hypoglycemic person.

For either person, the test should be before your first meal.

## *How Often to Test*

In starting out, I tested every day.  It is not easy to undergo a finger prick each day.  It takes about 12 minutes, with the preparation, the finger stick, and then waiting for the meter to give you a reading.  The preparation includes more than loading the injector with the lancet, and meter with the strip.  For me, it also meant warming my fingers, and shaking my hand to make it easier to get a sample of blood.  It takes several more minutes to record the reading, on a calendar, or a tablet/book.

Sometimes I made a quick analysis of why there was a change in my reading from the day before.  I found that I had to plan on 15-20 minutes for the test.  It is a small price to pay to avoid losing a leg, going blind, or early death.  At that time, it's then too late to wish you had taken the time to monitor your glucose level.  Once I was on the right path, and seeing my number going down, I gradually modified my program.  I started skipping the Sunday testing, and then sometime later, the Saturday testing, depending on the numbers, and the consistency of the numbers during the week.

In order to fight an enemy, you have to know the enemy.  You have to be able to see the enemy, among non-enemies.  You have to evaluate which enemies are the most threatening to you.

You, carrying out a self-help program, are in the best position to know this.  You will be collecting daily "scouting reports."  Thus is valuable information that your doctor doesn't have, when he sees you at several months' intervals.  Also, you will be reacting more quickly, as you see clearly, what food items are causing you to be a diabetic.

## *The Importance of Recording Test Results*

I began to visualize what information I needed, how to obtain it through testing, and how best to record it, in order to figure out what causes my blood sugar to go up or down. I decided that when you test, you should record the number, say on a large calendar used for just this purpose. Your test result may vary from the expected, and you will want to try to determine why.

The testing numbers will probably show an inconsistency, like:

| | |
|---|---|
| Monday | 131 |
| Tuesday | 143 |
| Wednesday | 125 |
| Thursday | 151 |
| Friday | 144 |
| Saturday | 133 |

The numbers jump up and down, all over the place. Remember they represent our current diet and lifestyle. By recording everything we ate or drank the day before, we will begin to know what affects our number. You may also want to record getting ready for, or having a stressful event. A possible recording is shown in Fig. 3. Using this type of recording is how I began a disciplined program to achieve a reduced glucose number.

| | Monday | Tuesday | Wednesday | Thursday | Friday |
|---|---|---|---|---|---|
| | 131 | 143 | 125 | 151 | 144 |
| Breakfast | Oatmeal, Raisins, Orange Juice, Coffee | Omelet, Toast, Decaf Coffee | Dry Cereal, Decaf Coffee | Oatmeal, Blueberries, Decaf Coffee | Omelet, Ry Toast, Deca Coffee |
| Lunch | Ham Sandwich, Milk | Pea Soup, Cola | Cheeseburger, Fries, Shake | Onion Soup, Salada | Tuna Salad |
| Dinner | Chicken, baked Pot, Salad, Apple Pie, Coffee | Salmon, Salad, Pie, Tea | Fried Chicken, Fries, Veggie, Grape Juice | Turkey, Peas, Beer | Steak, Potatoes, Green Beans, Bee |
| Snack | 10 p.m. – snack, nuts | | 10:15 p.m. cookies, review speech | | Peanuts at night |

**Figure 3**

In the example, on Tuesday, the glucose reading went up to 143 from Monday's 131. That meant that the person had to analyze what they ate, and when (snacks). This is how you learn what is happening to your body. I used this procedure to look at each day's breakfast, lunch, dinner, and snacks, and try to determine what caused changes to my glucose reading.

I hung a big calendar behind the bedroom door, and recorded the above type information on it. This is a very important part of the self-help approach. How else could I explain to myself, to others, including a doctor, as to what is causing me to have diabetes? In the military, it is called obtaining intelligence information, then analyzing it, and determining where and how the enemy is creating a threat that has to be counter-attacked.

It is interesting, challenging work, and a basic building block of the self-help approach.

## *Understanding Test Results*

One time, in recording my numbers for a week, they were 126-128-131-154-114. What was the difference between 126 and 154? I knew I was heading in the wrong direction. I was beginning to take supplements, and was modifying my diet.

In the sequence of 126-128-131, I felt I was getting there, although I didn't like the small up-hill trend.

The day before the glucose reading of 154, I enjoyed a new, very heavy carb meal. That pushed my reading up from 131. What to do? I decided to eat less carbohydrates, and achieved a drop of 40 points in one day. I went from a diabetic to a non-diabetic! My reasoning was less carbs would mean that there was less glucose from my body to process in one day.

A word of caution. I was a one day non-diabetic! When you are consistently below 120, or my goal of less than 110, you and I can say we are non-diabetic. Like a "recovering alcoholic", you may be a recovering diabetic, but you have to keep alert on your program, and be disciplined taking and recording your glucose level, recording your food, beverages, etc., and modifying your program where necessary.

Sometimes it is not easy to be disciplined. On a Tuesday that a good friend was opening a restaurant, my reading was 111. The next day it was 133! The culprit was jambalaya. I was pleasantly surprised to see it on the menu. Having been to New Orleans a number of times, I enjoyed this Creole dish of a large amount of rice, with shrimp, oysters, sausage, chicken, and spices. I was later to learn that the white rice was the culprit! It was a good lesson on the value of daily testing, and recording the result. On developing more understanding of diabetes, such as diet considerations, I was able to go back to my health history, and see cause and affect relationships more clearly.

We can't just always eat or drink everything that tastes good to us. On a very hot day, I noticed lemonade on the menu, in 16 oz. glasses. Two gurgled down easily. The next day, my number was way up. I forgot lemons are bitter, and for a nice tasting lemonade, you add a lot of sugar.

You too will develop a quizzical nature and will explore reasons why test results changes can occur day-to-day.

The day may come when you are in a consistent range of 103-105. Then one day, you see your reading at 134. Wow, is it threatening? Is it some unknown new enemy that is now going to do away with all the good thinking and discipline you have been achieving? No, it is a challenge! You need to backtrack and figure out what caused it, and then figure out what to change in the future. It is a challenge, not the time to go to the weeping wall with a poor-me attitude. It is an opportunity to reinforce that you are in control of your health.

Why can I say this? Because I lived it! Once I was in a consistent safe range, and then my glucose reading went way up. I was eating sweets, especially chocolate this and chocolate that. I then got back on my program. The next 8 days are my actual glucose readings. They are 139, 136, 126, 124, 115, 113, 108, and 101. When you have been in a disciplined program, and achieving results, then by analyzing your eating habits, and making a change(s), you can bring yourself back into a safe reading.

## _The Difference in Using the Fight Diabetes Program_

I was curious what treatment plan other diabetics were on, and how successful they were. In the last nine months, (sounds like a pregnancy), I have had discussions with many who were following the medicinal approach. I found that the treatment plan was usually a combination of having to take medicine to "control" the patients' glucose to an acceptable level, to "watch" their diet, and get more exercise. They were not given any specific information regarding diet or exercise, and very often were referred to a dietician. The doctor did not have the necessary background to go further in his advice to the patient.

In a way, this is similar to the dental community. A dentist, in evaluating what he sees in a patient's mouth may say, we need to fill this tooth, extract it, and so on. They would be focusing on the treatment, and not the cause. Many dentists will not try to determine how you brush your teeth, how often, and do you floss. They may not ask what sweets you eat, and how often, and do you have a filter on your water intake.

All of this would be helpful in helping patients change current habits to a more preventive set of habits.

The doctors' patients told me that their doctors usually prescribed taking 500 mg of Glucophage every day, for the rest of their lives.

Some doctors had little to suggest on a diet, except eat plenty of vegetables and fruits. This of course would include white rice, white potatoes, etc. They referred many patients to a dietician, and received the same general advice, without specifying what vegetables or fruits, and in what quantities.

Dr. Andrew Weil is quoted as saying, "The poor advice about diet and health that people get far too often when they ask physicians, nurses, registered dieticians, and other representatives of the health-care establishment for help, reflects the dearth of good nutritional education in our professional schools."

My primary physician is at Lahey Clinic and she alerted me to the possibility of diabetes. I have a profound respect for her, and for Lahey Clinic. It is one of the greatest diagnostic centers in the world. If a person has a medical problem, Lahey has a great ability to determine what it is, and what to do about it. They are not organized and equipped to understand, for all problems, how you got the problem in the first place. They can do some of this, but it is not in their area of strength. They also stress that they are not in the prevention end of the medical cycle, although they have some competence in this area. Lahey is the center of expertise for many medical problems, especially those of the heart. Diabetes is a fast growing problem without the research centers to back up the analysis needed to formulate a treatment.

Part of the difference in the Fight Diabetes Program is to focus on what is causing the diabetes in the first place. It gradually struck me that my objective was to determine why I, and others, "got" diabetes. That led me to use a scientific based approach to do my own research on the cause(s) of this dreaded disease. I developed hypotheses, sought expert inputs from on-going medical research, and then obtained data from testing, to verify the findings, or to discard them.

Many of the diabetic patients I talked with, told me that they were told to revisit the doctor every two to three months to check on their glucose level. In the Fight Diabetes Program, we can see the results of empirical testing by reviewing data from the "Test Laboratory", our body. This is another missing link in today's medical preferred treatment approach. We see the data quickly, as the patient reads their glucose level each day. By reviewing the prior day's eating, drinking, stress, and exercise, we can see the cause and affect relationships, of these factors on our glucose level. As the substitute doctor, we can analyze why our reading went up or down. For example, certain foods cause our bodies to raise our glucose levels. We adjust our diet, and observe the positive affect. We can also measure the affect of taking supplements. By maintaining the program over a period of time, we can see our body get to, and maintain a satisfactory glucose level.

The major difference in using the Fight Diabetes Program, and the current medical approach, is that the Fight Diabetes Program fills in the vacuum in the need for a program to stop creating, and continuing to create, diabetes at its source, in the first place. We don't gain an understanding of what is creating the enemy that we have to face, and defeat, by seeing a doctor every three months. It is also impractical for the doctor to see us every day. We can observe the impact of what we eat, drink, exercise, and think about day to day. We can adjust what we are doing daily, and this becomes our modified, practical, "treatment plan." We can review the results, say every three months with a doctor, and this is a more beneficial plan for us, and for our doctor.

By adhering to a program of supplements, using the Glycemic Index to select what foods to eat, and reducing the quantity of carbohydrates we eat by ignoring the low fat diet, and eating more protein, we can take the self-help approach to defeat diabetes.

## *Who is the Enemy?*

The American Medical Community, and perhaps others in the world, in the 1999 time frame, will tell any interested person, that diabetes cannot be cured. They will say, the cause of diabetes is a gene, a virus, or and accident/injury. They will prescribe medicine, usually glucophage, exercise, and say go see a nutritionist. There is an enemy, and the enemy can be overcome. As the comic character Pogo said, "we have met the enemy, and it is us."

Adult diabetics self inflict diabetes. It is what we put in our mouths, and how we use our minds.

- We eat and drink things that are not good for us.
- We are not able to eat some good things, like trace minerals, because they no longer exist, in sufficient quantity, to provide us with nutrients our bodies need.
- We react to happenings in our life by creating large doses of stress, which can increase glucose in our bloodstream, and this glucose is not utilized by our energy needs.
- We do not use our minds in a positive way, using meditation, and other ways of enhancing a stress-reduced state of mind.

Fight Diabetes Program provides a path for hundreds of thousands of adult diabetics to rid themselves of diabetes. Not everyone will try this path, and rid themselves of this dread disease. Not everyone will admit that they are causing their diabetes. They don't accept being personally responsible, and at fault.

It is easier to say that a gene is causing it, or they caught the flu and never fully recovered from it.

They may start taking a few supplements, perhaps a multi vitamin. There will be no appreciable, consistent change in diet. As they get progressively worse, they may scramble and at the last minute or two, try to get on a program, as they hurt too much, or fear death knocking on the door. Some will be in a long battle, for hopeful recovery.

Encourage as many as you can, as you experience your on-going recovery – which should be months, not years.

If this book is as successful as I think it will be, health organizations like the ADA, NIH, hospitals, physicians, HMO's, and others will begin to get the word out that the <u>Fight Diabetes Program</u> can defeat this killer, diabetes.

## _Validation of the Program_

In April 2001, I had my annual physical at Lahey Clinic. The results from my primary physician, as recorded in her official report, were –

| Reading | | Normal Range |
|---|---|---|
| Cholesterol | 183 | 130-200 |
| Glucose | 129 | 70-110 |
| HDL | 35 | 35-70 |
| PSA (prostate) | 1.1 | 00-6.5 |
| AST (liver) | 27 | 11-40 |
| ALT (liver) | 24 | 7-40 |

The glucose reading of 129 is the three month average.

After April 2001, I started the Reduced Carbo Diet.

I was seeing my glucose reading decreasing, now using this program, but I was wondering at what price.

Would I be endangering my heart? I needed verification on parameters such as cholesterol and blood pressure. I had data on my body from Lahey Clinic. It was almost exactly 7 months later in my physician's November official report. I was eager to make a comparison. I had been following a trial and error approach and had achieved moderate success in lowering my glucose reading in April to 129. In adding the Reduced Carbo diet, The Slow Digestion diet, and continuing the Supplements Program, I was starting to win the battle against diabetes.

I wondered, a little worried, in reducing my glucose level, would my cholesterol go way up, would I have heart problems? I had the means to make a comparison of the 11/10/01 and 04/12/01 data, and observe any negative results of eating eggs, red meat, etc., for seven months.

The following is a comparison between two sets of Lahey Clinic data.

|  | 11/10/01 | 04/12/01 |
|---|---|---|
| Cholesterol | 177 | 183 |
| Glucose | 99 | 129 |
| HDL | 31 (normal 40-75) | 35 (normal 35-75) |
| Ration chol/HDL | 5.7 (2-5) | 5.2 (2-8) |
| Triglycerides | n.a. | 55 (55-150) |

The answer to my concern, as stated above, is that my cholesterol went <u>down,</u> from 183 to 177. Eating more protein in the Reduced Carbo Diet was not endangering my heart, but reducing the danger of a heart problem. My blood pressure, as taken by a visiting nurse to the town, is essentially the same. My weight is the same.

My three-month average glucose reading had dropped 30 points! At a 99 glucose reading, it is well below ADA's safe reading of 120 and Lahey's 110. This is a highly respected national clinic verification of the success of the <u>Fight Diabetes Program.</u>

My HDL went down a little. I will find out what is needed to make it rise. I don't believe that HDL is a diabetic parameter of great interest. I will research this too.

Endorsement from experts or users of the <u>Fight Diabetes Program,</u> may give additional confidence that the program works. I used the scientific method, similar to a medical researcher, to develop the program, and then followed it. There is no question that it worked for me.

I now knew I was winning the fight. What a great feeling! There was more work to be done, as I wanted a continuation of reducing my glucose number, and maintaining a consistent safe number, but I could see victory over this silent killer just ahead.

## _Summary of Differences_

A silent killer named diabetes is on the rampage creating what the health authorities call an epidemic. It is not a true epidemic, like the plague, because it is not contagious. It is not transmitted person to person. We, ourselves, are the lone culprits. We do it to ourselves. It's like shooting yourself in the foot.

Due to a lack of nutritional training, most doctors do not have a medical base to help eliminate this disease. They are doing their best to prescribe how to control, or manage it.

"Insulin fails to prevent diabetes" was the headline for an article in a recent newspaper. "To doctors disappointment, a landmark study has found that preventive injections of insulin do not ward off a common form (insulin dependent) of diabetes. Doctors were already giving insulin to patients in the hope of preventing it." This is another example of the lack of the correct focus by the medical community, due to the lack of the correct, if any, nutritional training.

Their specialty is controlling the patients' diabetes, not getting rid of it or preventing it. As we have learned, prevention or elimination starts with what we put in our mouths.

Traditional treatment approaches apparently have not reduced the number of diabetics, significantly, or at all.

"_Winning the Fight Against Diabetes_" has promise of doing just that.

Doctors, like those who conducted the preventive injections of insulin research, should be encouraged to keep analyzing possible solutions to all of our medical problems. It would appear to be advantageous to cross link disciplines, such as medical diagnostics with nutritional preventive approaches. This could lead to significant new treatment programs.

This may also provide new "medicines" that are identified outside the research laboratories of pharmaceutical companies. Most, if not all, would become products of the pharmaceuticals, but better awareness of side affects may become known to the doctors.

There is a small paper that comes in the package of glucophage. It states "glucophage is not for everyone and may cause buildup of lactic acid in the blood, which is serious and can be fatal." I was not given this warning by the prescribing doctor. I feel doubly blessed in finding *"Prescription for Nutritional Healing"* which led to my using supplements, and in avoiding the possibility of a very serious side affect.

## *Additions to the Basic Self Help Program*

I discovered that there are other considerations that could help conquer diabetes beyond the basic nutritional program. Less important, but useful. Remember we are all different and I am not sure just yet how much more they can help us. But I would like to share some thoughts with you. Other diet considerations include eating, drinking, and cooking.

Recently, in some of the better health literature, I saw three recommendations regarding our diet. They are, (1) eat 5-6 meals/snacks a day, (2) chew your food, and (3) drink eight 8 oz. glasses of water daily. There is usually no stated reason for this. Interesting in that I feel all three can be related to diabetes. It all starts with too much sugar in the blood. We can also assume that the problem is too much sugar at a given point in time.

By spreading the intake of food/sugar, over a longer period of time, like 5-6 meals/snacks, with smaller portions, we give the body time to react to the input of sugar, and don't over-power our pancreas or our cells. It's the smaller portions, at any given time, that appears to be important here.

Chewing your food results in the same process, you spread the intake of food over a longer period of time. Chewing is the start of the digestion process. The saliva makes the food ready for our stomach to do its processing. Also, chewing makes each bite easy to swallow. In chewing, you give the saliva time to act on the food. Crushing and moistening food eases its trip to the stomach. Mothers know that it is easy to say, chew your food. Experience tells us that we need to have a procedure to make it happen. Try using counting. Count to 20-30 or so while chewing, and 7 or so, in-between mouthfuls. Our "Should do" statements are more effective if followed by a procedure, to make a desire into a reality.

There are many articles on drinking more water. Some of us may be at least partially dehydrated, without knowing this. This is very bad for our health. Yes, beer, wine, water in food all count, but look for easy ways to drink more water. Try taking a drink whenever you are in the bathroom or kitchen.

I consume at least 32 ounces of water each day, taking my supplements. You may want to fill a 16 oz. glass (not that big really) with water, and drink about a third of it before you begin with your first group. Throughout the day, divide your supplements into groups and take with 8 ounces of water.

I found a gem of information from the *"Sugar Busters Shoppers Guide"* (reading list), in their comment on cooking. They indicate that cooking raises the glycemic index of carbohydrates. It is therefore better to replace most canned carbohydrates with the fresh, dried, or frozen variety. It apparently is also true that cooking, especially overcooking, can cook out most of the nutrients.

When preparing your food, it may be best not to over-cook them, but cook them a la dente, or just a little firm.

Now that I had looked at what's best in eating slow digestion foods, downsizing the amount of a food being eaten, and adding protein to fulfill the appetite, it naturally lead me to try the prevailing wisdom of eating 5-6 meals/snacks a day. That sounds good, and it may work for many people. However, we are turning on the pancreas to generate insulin each time. Turning it on a large number of times meant I was depending on it to be a perfect pump.

For me, there came a gradual recognition, with everything else working in my disciplined program, that 5-6 meals/snacks or more, was just not working for me. Maybe the reason was that my body processes were too used to the traditional three meals a day. It doesn't matter; the reality was there that I needed another variation in my program.

It began with my morning meal. I usually had oatmeal three or more times a week for breakfast, and usually scrambled eggs or an omelet the other mornings. I ate either a single piece of toast, or none, no home fries, and no bagels, buns, or other baked goods. I also had a beverage before or during a meal, not after. This was for better digestion. Lunch was another light meal. By dinnertime, I was hungry, and ate a substantial meal. This seemed to work very well for me.

When going out to a very nice restaurant, and eating appetizer, soup/salad, entrée, and dessert, I had somewhat less than favorable results. The reading was higher the next day. This brings to mind our insulin generator pumping away all during the long time of the meal. It may be possible that it worked hard, but continued at a lower speed, so to speak, while waiting for the next entrance of food. There may be two things wrong with the prolonged meal. Once could be insulin is constantly being produced in different volumes, by our continuously-run pump, like a big and small stream of water coming out of our garden hose. This might cause the pancreas to cycle up and down, and even to shut down. It is interesting to note here that the pancreas has the ability to check on the amount of sugar in the bloodstream, acting something like a thermostat does. When needed, it generates insulin and sends it on its way.

This suggests that the day after a Thanksgiving type meal, my glucose meter might go off the scale. It's a little too early for me to confirm this affect of a large meal, with a long interval of time to eat it, to determine if it greatly hinders a sustained low glucose reading.

However, I am a believer that even if it does, an occasional special meal is probably good for us, instead of a continuous forced discipline. I wonder if there is something to the admonition, "Don't eat dinner, or snacks, late at night." By late, is usually mean too close to our bed times.

Is it possible that at nighttime, when our body functions start to slow down, that this includes our digestive system? If so, then the caution also relates to mitigating the threat of diabetes. The foods we have eaten could still be there, in our bloodstream, as sugar. Our pancreas slowed down, or called it a night. Sure the pancreas will start functioning when we eat in the morning. When we take our "fasting" reading though, we may have a high reading. In all probability, if this theory is right, we will probably have higher readings for a few days in a row. I just wonder about this.

I have not been recording my glucose levels many times a day, something like saving my fingers. Also, recording first thing in the morning seemed to give me a consistent basis, and one that was good enough to draw essential conclusions as to how my program was going.

The "don't eat late at night" concept may be a good reason to have our dinners at a reasonable time before retiring for the night, and also give up the munchies, crackers and cheese, etc. Whoever makes up the bed might agree. Other additions to the basic program include exercise, stress reduction, and using your mind.

## _Can Exercise Help?_

Exercise can reduce the amount of blood sugar circulating in your bloodstream. It may be a question of how much. Before analyzing that, let's understand that exercise has an added benefit. It can firm up, or build muscle. Women can benefit from muscle building without getting big and bulky. Check out women exercising in the local gym.

The key is that muscles are calorie-burners. Each pound of muscle burns up to 20 times more calories than each pound of fat. Strength training revs up our metabolism. There is an after-affect to strength training. Muscles continue to demand more calories to burn after the exercise.

We progress towards a more inactive society throughout the world, with more convenient and pampered transportation, TV entertainment, computer shopping, and so on, our daily activities now need less calories. However, most people would continue to consume the amount of food that they have become accustomed to eating. We need to be more active. Exercise classes and opportunities to be more active in our daily activities can all help. Exercise can be part of a diabetic prevention program, and also a program to rid yourself of diabetes. If you have diabetes, exercise does play a role. It's importance depends on what problem you are fighting. If you are 50 points or more above the safe level, you will need a lot of help in the form of a diet changes, and in taking supplements. Exercise probably plays a minor role. If you are 10-20 points above the safe level, either you have been doing a lot of things right, perhaps unknowingly, or the progression of your diabetes has reached a level where exercise is more important in halting the march to the serious complications.

All levels of exercise can be part of a diabetes care plan. Choose the type of exercise that you enjoy. It will have the best chance of making exercise into a routine. Good activities are walking, light aerobics, swimming, stretching, and strength training. The last two are especially important for seniors.

Regular activity improves blood flow, and blood pressure. It makes your heart and lungs stronger. This helps prevent the circulation and foot problems that people with diabetes can get. It also helps you handle stress better.

It has been stated that evidence is accumulating that the lack of exercise contributes to diabetes. A better perspective might be that being physically active lowers your blood sugar. It seems logical that exercise would help reduce the sugar in your bloodstream. The reason, exercise takes energy, to accomplish it. All energy comes from the cells. In order to move a finger, make a handshake, or exercise, our cells need to produce the energy that makes the physical motion take place.

OK, how does this happen? The cells produce energy by taking glucose (sugar) from the bloodstream, going past the cells "doors". The cells doors (receptors), open and receive the sugar, reducing the amount of sugar in the bloodstream. This then reduces your diabetes sugar count.

The cells "make" energy by burning the physical item, glucose, in their furnace. It's similar to burning wood in a fireplace, where a physical item, the wood, is converted to energy, heat and light.

My busy lifestyle did not leave me with time for exercise. This, of course, is the normal way of saying, even though I had 24 hours a day, I chose to spend my time doing other things. Being able to reduce my glucose level below 110, without any real exercise, is encouraging.

I do believe that a <u>regular</u> exercise program can reduce my, and your reading, at least another 10% or so. The key is to have a <u>regular</u>, consistent program. For example, if there is a quarter mile track near you at a high school or university, do not pat yourself on the back by going out and walking 6 times around (1.5 miles), once in a while. It may do you more harm then good. It is much more beneficial to do 2 laps, 3-5 times a week. Then build it up over several weeks to the 6 laps. The consistent exercise will allow your body to do you the most good.

## *The Impact of Stress and How to Combat It*

If we want to avoid diabetes, or get rid of it, we must think of it as another enemy we have to fight. I had heard of the "fight or flee" response, first described by Dr. Herbert Benson of Harvard.

It seems back in the caveman's day there were many dangers. A saber tooth tiger on the prowl could discover you. You say to yourself, I had better get out of here. You flee. Let's say you are in a cave with your family and an intruder starts to enter. You decide to fight him off.

In either case, in order to flee or fight, you need a burst of quick energy. You can't move your leg or arm without it. Where does the energy come from? It comes from your cells dumping glucose into your bloodstream and sending it on its way to feet, arms, etc. These cells need a continuous source of energy to fight or flee.

Now, lets fast-forward to today's environment. You get tense, agitated, or very upset over something. Your body reacts just the way it did hundreds of years ago. It deposits glucose into your bloodstream. Other than grinding your teeth, you are not doing anything physical to use up the glucose. Also, the pancreas sees no reason to send out insulin, so the glucose stays in your bloodstream to oxidize and become the dangerous free radicals.

The impact on your glucose reading is estimated to be about an 11% increase. You don't want to be injecting your bloodstream with unwanted glucose. The damage to your body depends on the frequency you become disturbed, and how long you remain in an agitated state. You need to develop coping techniques to limit the amount of damage you are willing to accept from the free radicals. You need to practice stress reduction.

I was surprised to learn that stress can produce hormones that can shoot our blood glucose levels up and out of our desired range. I found that I could eat the same diet, take the same nutritional anti-oxidants two days in a row, and have different glucose readings depending on the affect of a stressful event. Stress can be a hidden contributor to unexpected swings in blood glucose levels by 9-12 points. Relaxation techniques, meditation, massages, humor, are all helpful as reported in Prevention Magazine[3] and other periodicals. Also, don't fuss the little stuff; don't hold grudges, cut them some slack, etc. It also helps to develop a positive attitude. Whether at church or by yourself, massaging your spirit helps too.

Lets take a minute and go back to relaxation techniques. I have practiced relaxation techniques. To me, it meant developing specific techniques in order to be successful at relaxing. These techniques included learning to meditate.

Once relaxed, or in a state of meditation, there is always a choice between being passive or active. Passive means just relax and let the thoughts come to you. This is important in itself in that your body, in a relaxed state, is healthy.

When harried by the day's activities, a 15-minute passive relaxation period could be as beneficial as an hours sleep. A couple of these, now and then, even twice a day, will greatly help in reducing stress and in reducing glucose levels. I will discuss active relaxation/meditation in the section on using your mind. There are many good tapes that can help you develop meditation capability.

We should all learn that as babies, we breathed using our abdomen. Later in life, when the doctor asked us to take a deep breath, we inhaled into our lungs. Now, many practitioners of stress reduction and meditation are suggesting belly breathing. I have used the technique on occasion. It does quiet your system down. There are those who advocate training your system to belly breathe by spending a half hour doing this, now and then, so that it becomes a habit for your body. They maintain that it makes you healthier.

---

[3] Prevention April 2000 Edition, article on relaxation methods and benefits to reduce blood sugar.

Two years ago I was in a light aerobic class. This is an excellent way to reduce stress. There was an instructor, and we had a group of 25 or so – all in the same poor condition as I was. There wasn't time to think about yourself, as you had to concentrate on the desired movements of the exercise and rejoice when you were successful in doing them. There wasn't time to be thinking of the stressful events in your life.

A break in the program came, and I found myself with Ralph and a few others. Ralph was the oldest member by far at 87. Being curious, I asked him what he ate. He was perplexed, so I asked what he ate for breakfast. He said oatmeal and he cooked it himself, and threw in some raisins. "Okay, what else do you eat for breakfast?" "That's it, oatmeal." "Seven days a week?" "Yep!"

Jane, 74, overheard the conversation. "Me too," she said. "I was raised in an orphanage in Canada. We ate oatmeal every morning." I then decided to eat oatmeal more often. For example, in a favorite restaurant, I ask for a bowl of oatmeal, and a separate bowl of blueberries and walnuts. I knew blueberries were good for the diabetic and they enhanced the taste. I reasoned that if they had blueberry pancakes, they must be able to provide them as a side dish. I have since learned that oatmeal is too often an overlooked ally in helping adrenaline fight stress.[4]

Being curious about other people, such as I was with Ralph, is a great help in reducing, or even avoiding stress. Being genuinely interested in others is a great way to focus your mind away from yourself, and pre-occupy your mind in a positive way, and away from stress.

For those with hot tubs, or spas, I can pass on an interesting experience. I took my glucose reading as usual. Then at the urging of my wife, I soaked in the spa for about 15 minutes, which I rarely do. I was curious and took my reading again. It had gone down 5 points!

---

[4] Uncommon Cures for Everyday Ailments, Bottom Line

I don't know if this was practicing stress reduction, or that it was just a beneficial thing to do. If it works, it works.

It has been clear that we all have "incidents" that can cause us stress. Many of these are unavoidable. Some are somewhat self-induced. Those who naturally have a positive mental attitude, or who have cultivated it (using relaxation techniques, etc.), tend to attract less negative "incidents."

I have come to believe that those "incidents" that do penetrate our day-to-day existence, affect us to the degree we let them. It is our reaction to negative happenings that is the key. We will immediately produce a reaction, with a certain amount of our own negative energy. This will be a "spike" of energy. The amount of energy is what is important. If it is a very large amount, the amplitude of the spike will show the degree of physiological affects on our body. Our heart rate will increase, adrenaline will start flowing, and sugar will be produced (from fats) to allow us to respond and take physical action. It can be like a cook stove ready to explode. However, we can mentally adjust and shut it down. We can do this, incident by incident, or develop a demeanor that lets us control incidents, rather than them controlling us. There are some elder citizens I know that I believe have become quite expert at this.

The second important factor at work here is the duration of our reaction to the incident. Some people chew on the incident for quite some time. They have trouble letting it go. The longer we hold onto it, the more damage it can do to us.

The bottom line is you can affect your glucose level by how you react to incidents. These incidents can be stressful things to deal with in our relationships, family, friends, and career for examples.

Sometimes in a career, you can experience your boss taking over your creative idea, and presenting it as his or her own. You are understandably very upset. Now what?

Cycle down and demonstrate less creativity?  Go into a shell?  Go on the offensive and be secretive about your next creative idea?  How do you win?  How do you lose?

How do you lose is easy to see.  You build tension, which is harmful for the body in terms of diabetes, and other diseases of the body, when you turn negative.

It's tough when the natural reaction is akin to road rage.  Rather than reacting to someone invading your space, you virtually boil with the injustice of it all.

A tough call for handling negative incidents with a boss, or a radical driver, or any other relationship.  We all need to think it through and not just give in to a gut reaction.  Negativity generates more negativity.

With students shooting each other, instead of having fistfights, the schools are implementing new classes in "conflict resolution."  In going through the school of hard knocks, we need to develop coping techniques too.

That's how we win, as we expand our capabilities to deal with these stressful events.

It was reported that Paul McCartney was going through a difficult time.  He sensed the breakup of the Beatles was at hand.  It was also said that he was over indulging in booze and drugs.  He was in mental turmoil.

Paul often thought of his departed mother, but never could visualize her.  Then one night, he saw her face clearly when he was asleep.  She spoke to him and concluded with, Paul, <u>let it be.</u>

Paul carried that image and the words, let it be, with him the next day.  It inspired him to change his life.  He then wrote the song, "Let It Be" which has been an inspiration message for many.  Those who have heard it, used its meaning to relieve feelings of anger, frustration, disappointment, etc., over life's difficult incidents and its hard knocks.  It is an important message for all of us, and has a large potential to reduce the amount of stress we carry through life. I can see that let it be, is stronger than let it go. It's almost the difference between accepting the occurrence as part of our experience and relationships, and walking away from it.

Think about it! If the expression was "let it go", and we used it in our minds, to stop our conversation with another, instead of giving a rebuttal for one of their comments, then we walk away from the person, and the incident. But, we have not resolved it in our minds. It is still there, causing stress. If, on the other hand, we say to ourselves, "let it be", we take the ramifications of the incident into ourselves, deal with it, and it is done.

We can even smile to ourselves with this internal saying in its place. We are the better person, and interestingly, we are better off in having done this. And likely, we will learn from the experience. Practice collecting internal smiles.

Now, a different thought. Someone once said, "stressed" spelled backwards is "desserts." This point has some validity. We should reward ourselves for special moments, achievements, etc. You made something you were proud of. Celebrate!

You stuck by your diet, or diabetic program, and achieved positive results. Celebrate! You get the idea. Give your mind and your body some time to relax and celebrate life. It decreases stress.

You can't be happy and celebrating and stressed out at the same time. There is a residual benefit from being relaxed that carries itself forward. It may not result in a 24 hour or 7 day a week relaxation. But some relaxation will go forward and help you adjust to life's challenges.

I have learned these painful lessons. It was not easy with a redheaded temper, and an instant fight response. I am measurably better at it, but it is somewhat "a work in progress." It is more than procedural. You need to shift your value system.

We have talked about our one-on-one situations. What about you on you? How we live our lives can have a major impact on stress. Many people are helter-skelter busy. There is not enough time to do everything we would like to do. We multi-task like crazy people. It can be said that our heads are full of mental muck. We need to adopt the strategy of first things first, and one thing at a time. We have to also add some quiet time to our agendas. Not when we can get to it, but planned quiet time.

If stress causes a higher reading and if this is because sugar does not exit from our blood easily, or if there is a reduction in the production of insulin because of the stress, is there a cellular process that causes this? If this cause and affect relationship is known explicitly, then maybe there is a way to mitigate stress's impact on us. This may be of interest to the NIH cellular research labs. Maybe technology can save us, but let's do what we can do to prevent big gobs of stress by how we live our lives.

"Whatever the mind of man can conceive and believe, it can achieve."
Napoleon Hill

## *Your Mind is Part of Your Fighting Equipment*

Using one's mind to either stay healthy, or to resolve one's problem is definitely in. There are many books that address this. Some are shown in the Reading List, including Joan Borysenko's *"Minding the Body, Mending the Mind"*, Jose Silva's, *"The Silva Mind Control Method"*, and Norman Cousins's, *"Anatomy of an Illness."* These and other authors have proven the value of using your mind to combat diseases.

A very simple technique is to talk to your mind. Yes, your mind listens and responds. Not always in the direct manner you may expect of another, but very often in the best way. I know that for some it is a practice they have developed that is very effective for them. You can learn and practice affirmations daily. A very famous doctor in France, Emil Coue, has popularized this technique. He taught his patients to say, "Day by day, in every way, I am getting better and better." It worked, as he observed some of his patients that did this show very impressive improvements.

Tell your body you want to get rid of diabetes, believing that it will. You may be surprised if your body talks back to you, most likely in the form of a thought during the day.

Relaxation and meditation techniques may be effective auxiliary forces to help you in your fight against diabetes. You can learn and practice relaxed states of mind and meditation.

It is complicated and may not appeal to many. However, it is very effective for some. It is said that the great golfer, Jack Nickalaus, improved his golf game using these techniques. You can learn relaxation techniques that allow you to go into a meditative state. When in a meditative state, we can make it a dynamic, rather than a passive experience. We can practice visualization, and imagination. Visualization can be seeing a bicycle, in all of its parts.

You can project your visualization on a screen in your mind, and see the handlebars, wheels, etc. This ability to visualize is something that can be very helpful for your general health, and it comes easier with practice. Now, if we want to use our imagination to see the wheels on the bicycle are moving, that is the further development of our dynamic mental experience. These dynamic techniques are now being taught to cancer patients. The patients are taught to develop an image of the disease. This is visualization. The patients are then taught to see their body fighting the disease, using the dynamic image they have created. There is a case where a female patient put herself on her screen, on a beach, where she was being chased by a dark figure, her image of her cancer. The patient saw herself in a contest with the dark figure. She jumped into the water and swam to an island, beating the dark figure to it. This created the feeling that she could beat her cancer. Using our dynamic mind to fight a disease can be a helpful addition to a patients basic program.

For diabetics, when in a meditative state, there could be many, but each personal, dynamic creation. Perhaps an insulin-dependent diabetic could visualize an old pump that was no longer working effectively, and taking it to a store and trading it in on a brand new one. Perhaps a non-insulin diabetic could create a butler/waiter to escort the glucose to a room where there would be a warm welcome, a reception by the cell receptor, so to speak. We are all creative and can create a personal image that will work for us. It will take practice in developing our capabilities. We will never know when we <u>have</u> to use this tool. In the meantime, we can use visualization and imagination techniques in winning over diabetes.

Maintain a positive attitude. Reduce anxieties by avoiding stimulants. Exercise can take your mind off a lot of mental processing. I intend to start a regular exercise program and reduce my number further. Seek out the benefits of a mind-body partnership.

## *The Battle is Won*

The week my glucose reading was consistently in the range of 103 to 108, I felt that warm glow flow over me. I had won the battle to rid myself of diabetes!

The dedicated, tireless pursuit of this silent killer had been worth it. Reading medical research from around the world, analyzing it, discarding some, and using some, has proven its worth. Knowledge is king!

Using the ever-changing database to modify my diet, and the taking of the supplements, developing practices of the mind, beginning to exercise, using stress reduction techniques, had all lead me to that plateau of being free of diabetes.

The specific supplements at the right dosages had provided me with fighters that in numbers and in combination could defeat hungry free radicals feasting on my inner body.

That was not the end of the battle, as the wrong diet I was eating was generating more free radicals with every spoonful of the wrong diet, or gurgle of the wrong beverage. These were new fighters, and as the fallen free radicals were dragged off the battlefield, our weary and outnumbered fighters had to mount a charge to counter the new free radicals. I needed my slow digestion diet, and reduced carbo diet to keep from creating a new group of the enemy.

There were other additions to the basic program that enabled my body to get below a reading of 110, my goal. There will be some who will find some of these additions to be very significant portions of their program.

The hunt is over. The fight continues day-to-day, to maintain the hard ground that has been won. After awhile, it becomes fairly routine.

It follows that I was compelled to write this book so that others can follow and rid themselves of diabetes. It's time to celebrate! You, because you now have a path, and me, because I have already followed the path.

My relatives and friends now have an opportunity to start down the path to rid themselves of diabetes. I want them to be successful. I no longer want to feel their pain, and see the fright in their eyes. Some have started on the path, and are achieving positive results. They are not there yet, but I look forward to their victories, step by step.

My fond hope is that others, in America, in the world, will find this path to rid themselves of diabetes, or to prevent it.

Remember, whether you are accomplishing ridding yourself of diabetes, or preventing getting diabetes, your goal should be to achieve this! But also remember, a goal, without action, is only a wish.

## *Other Diabetic Programs*

In addition to providing the nutritional approach that I followed, with success, it should be recognized that there are other programs that can be helpful. They include medicine that usually provides at least some degree on control, if not elimination of diabetes.

Also, I know someone who is utilizing a homeopathic approach, to maintain his glucose in a controlled state, instead of taking medicine. Recently, dispensing the standard "remedy" has been augmented to include supplements.

Even though this book reports on the experience of an adult-onset diabetic, in ridding oneself of diabetes, some of the Fight Diabetes Program should be beneficial to the juvenile. There is also a benefit to the non-diabetic in developing a preventive program from the information presented here.

Having accumulated extensive nutritional knowledge, and understanding of the body processes, I could see where there could be a missing diagnosis of one having diabetes, without the medical community being aware of it.

My objective was to rid myself of diabetes, to defeat the disease that now existed in my body. I was very successful in developing fighters (specific supplements), to go forward and defeat the enemy. I then had to identify the cause of the diabetes, and find a way to eliminate it through proper diet. It is a solid program.

We will look at other programs that are of value. They include –

Homeopathic medicine

Help for the juvenile diabetic

And

Prevention program for the non-diabetic

A count gram and low frequency eating programs

We will then look at the possibility of those who the medical community states are not diabetic, but I believe they could be.

That will get us to what we can do to help others who are already seriously wounded in their battle with the enemy. We will look at those who have two of the serious complications of diabetes, neuropathy and macular degeneration. They are facing possible loss of limb or eyesight.

## _Homeopathic Medicine_

I explored homeopathic medicine as an aid to eliminating diabetes. A friend had used it to go from a glucose level above 200, to one below 120. After being in the program for a few years, he has added many of the supplements that I was taking. Based on what he told me, I feel that the major improvement was attributed to his homeopathic treatments. My initial visit cost was around $250, with follow up visits around $85.

As I understood and experienced it, the key for the practitioner in solving the need for homeopathic medicine, was to interview a "patient" to determine what was at work in their sub-conscious mind. That was to be the source of the diabetic problem. A difficult concept to accept, but I tried to go down that path with the practitioner. I never achieved the dramatic results of my friend. As my already established program continued, I could see that I was making progress with it, and my visits with the practitioner kept getting further, and further infrequent, and I gave them up. The results were not worth the expense to me, in my fight to rid myself of diabetes.

It evidently works for some, but the psychoanalysis interviewing of the initiate, may be just window dressing. The real essence could be the giving of a "remedy." The remedy, like getting a shot, is pre-determined to correspond to the need for a particular health problem. The remedy was taken from a remedy box and given to me to swallow. There was no mixing of a new item from basic materials.

The remedy followed the rule of "similars", by taking a small dose that produces a small reaction similar to the health problem, and thus this gives the body the opportunity to fight off this problem. In so doing, the body's systems are activated to fight off the larger health problem. Something like that. It was never really explained to me. This method of treatment seemed to be based on a great deal of research, a "try it and see approach", that developed the remedies.

The whole approach seemed to be diagnostic medicine that followed a path of described problem (diabetes) to a treatment (remedy) to remove it. It was not an analysis as to how one gets the health problem in the first place. That is, until you add in the interview process, which for me, never led to an explanation of why diabetes was now occurring, or even a logical explanation of why the remedy. As I say, it evidently works for some, and I invite a close scrutiny of the reference in the reading list. It may very well be worth trying, for some.

## *Help for the Insulin Dependent Diabetic*

Let's talk first about obtaining help that could be beneficial.  Then let's look at preventing the problem in the first place.

Most of the information presented so far is focused on helping a non-insulin dependant diabetic.  Even though my journey has identified a program for those who are non-insulin dependent, I would like to pass on, what knowledge I have obtained.  If this helps anyone who is leading less than a full life, I will be happy.

The same suggested supplements and diet approaches for non-insulin users might also be effective for insulin users.  For example, Dr. David D. Williams, of "Alternative" reports that "Diabetes Care" stated in one of their issues, that a study found that 600 mg of alpha lipoic acid (ALA), taken twice a day, similar to the Fight Diabetes Program, can significantly reduce the need for insulin.  Also, ALA increased insulin sensitivity.

If you have to take insulin, it usually means that your pancreas is not producing enough insulin.  You need to take insulin shots to supplement what your pancreas produces.

From what we have learned so far, it would seem logical if there is only a small amount of insulin being produced in your body, then only a small amount of carbohydrates should be eaten, and they should be of the slow digestion type.

In my research, I have uncovered some specific approaches, for the insulin-dependent diabetic that could be helpful.  There are some experts who believe the bay leaf can extend by months, the time one can avoid insulin shots, or at least minimize reliance on shots.

You can steep several bay leaves in hot water, for a tea to be taken as 2-3 cups a day.  Maybe it's worth trying for a weekend.  Record the results each day.  Be careful; never eat the leaves as a shortcut.

In what might be a very desirable operation, but also a very expensive one, Dr. James Shapiro of the University of Alberta in Edmonton, Canada, has transplanted islet cells. These are the cells in your pancreas that produce insulin. If some of your insulin-producing cells have been destroyed, this replacement process may be of high interest.

This procedure evidently frees patients from their need for insulin shots. A chance to start over in life. The NIH and the Juvenile Diabetes Research Foundation are funding ten centers to conduct more research on the procedure. This would appear to be worthwhile to watch with the expectation that a more economical procedure could emerge.

Equally interesting is the work of Dr. Denise Faustman, of the Massachusetts General Hospital, as reported in *"Diabetes Interview"* (reading list). In her laboratory, she and her staff have injected live, healthy, <u>spleen</u> cells; from healthy non-diabetic mice into type 1 diabetic mice. The spleen cells were then turned into islet cells that produced insulin. This experiment completely and permanently reversed the diabetes in the type 1 mice – even in those mice that were close to death.

The focus of the experiment was to address the autoimmunity problem of diabetes. The researchers were amazed that the pancreas spontaneously regenerated itself, once autoimmunity was resolved.

We have learned that the pancreas produces insulin. It follows then, if we can do anything to help the health of the pancreas, it just might be able to produce more insulin.

Dr. James Balch recommends bean pot tea, made up of beans (kidney, white, navy, lima, and northern). The tea detoxifies the pancreas. Cedar berries are also excellent nourishment for the pancreas. Also huckleberry (bilberry) helps to promote insulin production.

The ayurvedic remedy, Gymnema Sylvestre, can be helpful for both dependent and non-dependent diabetes. It appears to stimulate the pancreas to produce more insulin, and to enhance the activity of insulin. Maybe it's like swimming upstream better. Typical dosage of 400 milligrams per day is recommended.

An ancient Greek and Roman remedy, Fenugreek, has been used to treat diabetes by lowering blood glucose. Non-dependent users are reported taking about 5,000 milligrams of powdered seed a day. It also comes in 500 mg tablet form. Dependent users are taking 8 to 10 times that amount. I would be more inclined to take 500 mg twice a day. Various health magazines have begun to tout this old time remedy.

Eating plenty of raw fruits and vegetables is stated as reducing the need for insulin. Exercise produces an insulin-like affect in the body. This may be why some diabetic athletes reduce their insulin dosage before exercise, or an athletic event.

Do not take cysteine; it can interfere with absorption of insulin by the cells. Also, do not take extremely large doses of vitamin B1 (Thiamine) and C. Excessive amounts may inactive insulin. The Balch recommended amounts are okay.

Harvey and Marilyn Diamond state that cow's milk, intended for young cows, has a protein that results in adding a coating to a human's beta cells. This essentially causes the cells destruction.

As we grow older, we tend to drink less milk. The Diamonds, in their books, *Fit For Life*,[5] (reading list), saw the potential danger of cow's milk in their book in 1985, and advocated giving it up when the young child started walking. The Diamonds pointed out that the chemical composition of cow's milk is different from that of human milk. The enzymes necessary to

---

[5] Fit for Life I and II, Harvey and Marilyn Diamond, Warner Books

break down and digest milk are rennin and lactase. In most humans, these digestive processors are all gone by the age of three.

This lack of processing in the human body leads to various problems in the body. As the latest research suggests, it could lead to the loss of beta cells. The deduction of the research is that cow's milk is the main cause of insulin-dependent diabetes. It would be surprising if the milk industry were not following this research. Perhaps their solution is to add the missing, necessary ingredients, to the milk.

What this suggests to me at this point in time, is for mothers to try to wean their babies as long as possible, to get them to where they can take regular food. This also suggests that perhaps adults should greatly reduce the amount of dairy products they eat. For diabetics, like any other treatment approach, a try it and see plan with careful monitoring of any short term and long-term changes in glucose, is warranted.

In summary then –

- It is obvious that reducing the load on our pump, the pancreas, could be beneficial. This depends on whether there is still a capability left in the pancreas. If we can assume there is some capability, the diets, slow digestion and reduced carbo, become very important in our body's utilizing whatever quantity of insulin is available, in processing glucose into the cells.

- Supplements can help, especially ALA, Gymnema, fenugreek, and zinc and other trace minerals.

- Certain food preparations such as bay leaf tea, bean pot tea, and eating bilberry and cedar berries, and raw fruits and vegetables, are also beneficial for the insulin-dependent diabetic.

- Maintain at least a modest, sustained, exercise program.

- Have caution regarding the drinking of cow's milk and eating cheese products, especially from the age of three on. See *"Fit for Life"* in the Reading List, if you would like more information on this subject.

- There is interesting technology being developed, thanks to the medical community. This includes transplanting new, healthy insulin producing cells. We need to be cautious and monitor the results of the research carefully. The same thinking goes with the injection of live spleen cells. It has worked for mice, now let's see if it works for humans. It's ok to be optimistic.

## *Junior*

I met Junior when I gave his Dad a copy of the book. Junior was a baby boomer gaining experience to take over Dad's business, when the time comes. Junior was a diabetic. He was an insulin dependent diabetic! His glucose reading ("the number", as we all call it) was in the hundreds. He said his body no longer produced insulin. He took carbohydrates by the number of grams he was to eat. After eating, he injected the required insulin for that number of grams. A very automated procedure. He was a little thin under his business suit. He said he was used to eating one meal a day, and that was a very large one. We had about a ten-minute conversation.

With injections of insulin, his "number" was in the 160-170 range. He was pleased to be "controlling" it. I gave him a copy of my first book. He wanted my phone number so that he could call if he had any questions. Stop reading this and think about it as someone who has read this book, and has an understanding of what I was thinking when talking to Junior.

Just think about it yourself, applying what you have learned in the book, as to what the problem is, and how can it be handled. Then read on.

One thing that Junior should discover is that as long as his "number" is above 120, he will have glucose in his bloodstream that is oxidizing and free radicals are attacking various tissues in his body and he will start to get the serious complication of diabetes.

A second thought that should come to you is there is no selection process of what is ok to eat and what isn't. There were no concepts such as the slow digestion diet, the reduced carbo diet, etc. There is not telling how much food he is actually eating and what food he is eating.

Now let's think about him saying, "my body no longer produces insulin", i.e. that his inslet cells have died. Did they, or does he have that elusive "insulin resistance" that the medical community is now using, or possibly neither? Place your bets.

The cause of inslet cells "dying" is usually given as a virus, or an injury. My guess is that as an adult, you do it to yourself. Maybe wrong, but let's try this hypothesis and see. I lean toward insulin resistance rather than cells dying. Back to the "Thanksgiving" meal way of eating. A very large meal takes a long time to eat. Can't you just see him, eagerly awaiting his one very large meal of the day, and probably washing it down with a suitable beverage? He then repeats this, day after day. For this large meal, there is a continuous stream of glucose going into his bloodstream, and his insulin is trying to match up with it. Given that this occurs, the insulin tries to get the cells open to receive the glucose. At some given point, it must be that the cells refuse to open their "doors", as they are full. This I would accept as insulin resistance and it would seem logical that it does happen.

I would suspect that the pancreas has a way of knowing that there is still too much glucose in the bloodstream. The only remedy that it knows is to produce more insulin and send it into the bloodstream.

Can it be, that the pancreas, the poor overworked pump, shuts down? Then it would not be a case of inslet cells dying, or the entire fault of the cells resistance, but a pancreatic failure.

If Junior were to spread out five or more small meals a day, align his diet with the Fight Diabetes diets, and take the recommended supplements, would you bet on an improved number? By improving the intake process, there should be some gain. My advice to Junior is to do the above but continue to take his insulin shots. If he notices he doesn't have to take as much insulin as before, he would so advise his doctor and go on a program of less insulin, and give up measuring the amount of carbohydrates.

Oh yes, the pancreas pump. With an improved intake process, we would like to see improved internal processing. The pump has not had an opportunity to demonstrate it is still functioning.

It either has nothing to process, or is overwhelmed by the "Thanksgiving" meal. It is not working during the fasting periods, and is not known if it is working during the big meal, as the insulin injection follows. It probably is still functioning when given the chance with the spaced out small meals.

This diabetes is a fascinating study, is it not?

## *If Non-Diabetic, Adopt a Prevention Program*

The key is that you will have to start taking charge of your health. Don't let your life just drift along, and one day wake up with diabetes.

Let's start off with a simple prevention activity. Exercise can be helpful. Remember, every time you move part of your body, your cells will open and send out energy in that part of your body that needs the energy. Then your cells want more glucose to be able to convert it into energy for a future need. If you are running away from a black bear, you don't want to run out of energy. The goal of exercise should be to match the intake of glucose.

The cells that just burned up some of their stored glucose, will look to take in glucose circulating in your bloodstream in from of their "doors", thus reducing the free radicals.

This is only a small part of a non-diabetic practicing prevention. The real essential part starts with the finger prick test. There are six basic test sets. I started with one of the six test units. I now use One Touch Ultra. Only 1 ul amount of blood is needed, whereas up to 4 times that amount is needed by other kits. All are needle systems, but this one is much less painful. If the reading is over 120, the person should get on the Fight Diabetes Program.

If below 120, start a prevention program. First, test on an empty stomach. Second, test 2-3 times a week. Record the test readings and what you ate or drank, etc. Monitor the results – play doctor. Then start a simple regimen of essential supplements, but at a prevention level, not a treatment level. For example, ALA could be 200 mg not 600, chromium 200 mcg not 500, carnitine, glutamine, and taurine one 500 mg a day, biotin 30 mg not 50, zinc 50 mg not 80, and continue with less dosage amounts about 1/3$^{rd}$, for the other supplements.

Sooner or later, as we age, the body needs help in taking in metals such as zinc, manganese, and magnesium. It matters like if the reason is metabolic reason of age, or lack of the mineral in the soil. Deficiencies in these can lead to diabetes, regardless of what you eat/drink, and what, if any, exercise. Adding manganese, say 5 mg, and magnesium 300 mg, along with zinc 50 mg, may prolong your need for a treatment program.

The key is to self-test to see if you have edged into becoming a diabetic. You can't wait for your occasional checkup, or in not having any checkup. Your body needs certain supplements as you age, and it is good medicine to start adding them for diabetes prevention, and for your general health. You should test your glucose reading once a month to see if you are becoming a soon-to-be-diabetic. If not, great! You are doing many things right. If you are becoming a diabetic, start a prevention program. Change your monitoring program to every two weeks. If you need further help in avoiding the serious complication of diabetes, start the total <u>Fight Diabetes Program.</u>

Let's summarize –

- Prevention is important. There is an old saying, "an ounce of prevention is worth a pound of cure".

- Over a million Americans are diagnosed each year as having diabetes. They didn't know that they had it. Remember, it is a silent killer, with none of the usual symptoms of a problem inside you. Also, you can go on leading a rather normal life, and not know you have diabetes.

- As we age, we incur deficiencies in trace minerals, such as zinc, that are important to our health. These deficiencies can lead us to diabetes. It is not a case of the body no longer having the ability to absorb these essential items from the vegetables we eat. They are diminishing in the soil in which vegetables are grown.

- You need to self-test, a few times a week, using the Self-Test procedures that have been presented to you. You may want to start taking some supplements.

- You are providing some of the activities that a doctor and nurse do. The real important fact is that you must step forward and take a significant role in maintaining your good health.

## *The Don't Eat Much Diet*

We have free radicals swarming around in our bloodstream and then attacking our bodies. We suffer the serious complication of diabetes. We take in supplements, and these fighters take on the free radicals in a battle, and it is a battle we can win.

The problem is that more free radicals can be coming and it becomes a continuous battle to see whether we have more of our fighters than the free radicals. Where are they coming from? As the leader of our defensive army, we know that they are a result of what we eat and drink.

We have learned to eat low glycemic index foods that allow our pancreas to produce insulin to keep up with then newly digested food, now glucose. This match up works on the battlefield. The interesting question is, will a low quantity of food also work? Let's look at the 220 gram program, and then the low frequency program.

## *The 220 Gram Program*

This is the story of Al, a good friend. At the time I was almost complete on the writing of this book, Al and I were having a cup of coffee together. We started talking health. He was very interested in the messages in my book, as he had read a copy of the manuscript. He agreed that medicine and exercise were not the essentials in ridding oneself of diabetes. He did feel that carbohydrates were the key.

His approach I would call the Super Discipline Approach. Mentally, he is very capable of following a program of this type. He limits himself to 220 <u>grams</u> of carbs a day!

He follows the Glycemic Index in a casual way. He only eats 220 grams of carbs a day and he knows exactly what he eats, and the number of carbs in each food item. He says that he is under the 120 glucose reading number.

Let's reason this out. First, if it works, it works. For how many people? It must be those persons with a very strong ability to discipline themselves. Second, you have to analyze every meal or snack in advance and know the total grams of carbs that you are consuming. Sound similar to Junior? The difference is that Al is not going to inject himself with insulin to meet the needs of glucose generated by the food he just ate. He is not going to need much insulin with a 220 gram carb meal. This would seem to have added success if he were eating slow digestion foods. With a very limited amount of carbs, there is very limited work for the pancreas to put out in insulin into the bloodstream. It follows that there would not be any insulin resistance. The cells are not being bombarded with lots of insulin to take in the glucose in the bloodstream and to process it. There could be a very good match between the amount of glucose and the amount of insulin needed to process it.

It works for him, but there may be a small percentage of people who will follow it because of the strict discipline required, and the detailed knowledge of the number of grams one is eating. There might very well be a sense of boredom with this method of eating as well. Some may want to try it, and it may work for them.

## *Low Frequency Eating Program*

If we look back to grandfathers of grandfathers, and beyond, we will probably see nomadic tribes moving around, hunting for food. When they could find some, they then ate. This was an original low frequency eating program, but not by choice.

Lately, there have been stories in the newspapers that say that people that eat less, live longer. Other stories say that on-going research supports this. Rose Kennedy, mother of John, the president, was asked in her 90's what she attributed to her long life. "I don't eat much" she replied. According to Oreste D'arconte, the theory is that caloric restriction holds back the aging process by altering our metabolic functions. There could be merit to this thought. Metabolism is the complex physical and chemical processes involved in maintaining life. Some may want to try to make some adjustment in their life styles.

For us fighting diabetes, there will be some like Al, who may want to follow a very restricted quantity of food approach, and others, an approach to delay aging. It would appear the construction worker, and other large users of energy in their bodies, would need the energy that our cells deliver from processing the glucose. They need a quantity of food that matches up with their energy needs. This then brings us back to the quality of the food, the glycemic index.

There is also the habit of three meals a day. This is far from the hunter-gatherer way of life. Maybe by reducing one or more meals, and going to snacks, is something to experiment with. For some, eating less frequently is an economically forced way of life. Others may want to adapt their life style to follow a low frequency program, at least to some degree.

To sum this up, you will need to take supplements to fight your fight, either to rid yourself of diabetes, or to prevent diabetes. You can modify your diet to the reduced carbo diet, and the slow digestion diet, or you can try a major life style change.

## *When is a Non-Diabetic a Diabetic?*

This chapter of the book has the potential of helping millions of people, perhaps around the world, who are really diabetic, and nobody knows it. This includes their doctor. Who are these millions? They are the people whose normal amount of glucose in their bloodstream is fairly low. It should be near a reading of 70 milligrams per deciliter. They are hypoglycemians (hypos) as contrasted with hyperglycemians (hypers), whose normal should be around 120.

Let's go slowly here. There are two dangers if you are a hypo. The most common danger is one of immediate concern. It is when the hypo goes below the 70 mg/dl. There is not enough glucose circulating in the hypos bloodstream. Because glucose is the most very important nutrient for the brain, a deficiency will cause problems. These can be dizziness, blurred vision, confusion, coma, and death. The remedy is to ingest sugar, like a candy bar.

The other danger is more long term and represents the condition of exceeding the 70 mg/dl by a significant amount, repeatedly. When this happens, the hypo can experience the same free radical affects on their body as a hyper could. There are several hypos, I know, who feel content with a glucose level of 90, not realizing the danger.

I feel that hypos need to have their glucose reading tests interpreted as to how close they are to their "normal" reading of 70. No different than a hyper wanting to know how close he or she is to 120. Nobody is aware that some hypos are diabetic because the usual medicinal approach is to test to see if everyone's (hyper or hypo) glucose reading is between 70 and 120. If so, the conclusion is that you are not diabetic. And the patient being tested is no way the wiser. The hypos with the abnormal readings are left ignorant of their impending peril.

These hypos may have been eating the wrong food, and drinking the wrong beverages most of their lives. They may have neuropathy, eye problems, kidney problems and their doctors will not know the cause. Because some may be poor and have to eat the wrong foods, some doctors will

142

identify the problem as family genes.  Everybody eating white bread, white rice, etc., does not a gene problem make.  It is an environmental, not a heredity problem.

Okay, let's ask the question – when is a non-diabetic, a diabetic?  Remember the person the doctor said had all of the symptoms (neuropathy, macular degeneration, etc.) but not the important one of a glucose reading above 120?  If not above 120, the doctor will say that the patient is not a diabetic.  It's as simple as that, or is it?

Based on his diagnosis, I would have thought it more correct if the doctor had simply said that the patient does not have an <u>elevated</u> glucose reading.  The real diagnosis is whether it <u>really</u> is a case of an elevated reading!

Let's remember that most health organizations, use "a normal range of 70-120", as the standard for determining a diabetic.  It's clear to see that a person with a glucose reading of 140, where "normal" is 120, is a diabetic.  Free radicals are causing damage in their body.  It would seem logical then, that a hypoglycemic person, who usually has a low concentration of glucose in their blood, with their reading normally around 70, with a reading of 90, also has an elevated glucose level 20 points above their normal.  This person IS a diabetic, and should be given a treatment plan that addresses the progressive deterioration of their limbs, eyes, heart, etc!


This can be illustrated as below –


```
_____ /////_____ /////_____

70        90                    120          140
```

Let's not look at a reading, of say 90, as being in a safe range of 70-120, but as a variance from the norm for that person. Let's stop diagnosing and obtaining readings that are observed in a range, that a nurse is trained to read as normal. Let's have physicians first establish a variance around 70, and a variance around 120, as a better means of determining whether a person is diabetic and should be given a treatment plan that helps the newly identified diabetic.

The Fight Diabetes Program would be applicable to them too! Who needs progressive neuropathy bad enough to have a leg amputated?

Doctors may decide to treat hypoglycemia patients as diabetics, based on the premise above. This is when the patient's glucose reading is significantly above their normal glucose reading of around 70 or so. They may advise the patient to use the full program as described in this book, in order to give patients the chance to rid themselves of diabetes.

If doctors do not advise patients to do so, there is a compelling reason to at least put into practice a portion of the program. Something is causing neuropathy, macular degeneration, etc., for those labeled non-diabetic. Those in the medical community that I have talked with do not know the cause. I have asked neurologists what causes neuropathy, and have been told that they do not know. I have asked eye specialists a similar question about macular degeneration, and received the same answer. Let's assume that it is our old enemy, free radicals. There is much to gain in trying to eliminate the free radicals.

The answer then, is to fight the free radicals with anti-oxidants. We identified those fighters in the section on supplements. Patients who can be identified as hypos, with variances, should also begin to take the recommended diets, to slow down, or prevent serious problems.

The sad thing is that many will not take action to help themselves rid themselves of diabetes. A primary reason is that these "hidden" diabetics do not want to go against the medical establishment. They have been raised to believe that doctors are like god. They are infallible.

Many of the doctors now know that they are not god-like. They can only perform from their basis of knowledge. That basis is changing drastically as more research proves old theories, and procedures, wrong. It has been a case of not really knowing, and therefore having to make the best judgment that they could. Many persons have started to say, "Hey doctor, (or a famous expert), last year you told me so and so, and now you are telling me something different. I don't know what to believe."

It will take readers of this book; patients and doctors, to explain the above need to not test to a range, but to test to the standard for hyperglycemia and hypoglycemia. Patients will only be able to penetrate the unknowing to a limited degree. It will take the doctors, and associations like ADA, NIH, and World Health to get the message out. It is particularly hoped that the ADA will recognize value in this new approach and start to use its resources to spread the word to adult onset diabetics. The insurance companies, the veterans organizations, Senior Groups, the Rotary, and many world health organizations, can cause a significant new enrollment of diabetics, but they will be getting the proper treatment to avoid amputation, blindness, heart attacks, and the other serious complication of diabetes. This "silent killer" will now be in the open, to be attacked.

## *Dave*

I met Dave at a meeting in a neighboring town hall. We were in the corridor waiting for a meeting to start. I initiated a social conversation. Dave started talking about his lifestyle. He said he was taking medicine, ate carefully and was trying to keep his glucose reading around 95. With a target of 95, I guessed he was a hypoglycemia. He said he was. He then said he was a diabetic. It was like finding a white rhinoceros walking down your street.

I was astonished that as a hypoglycemia person, he would identify himself as diabetic! He was under a doctor's care and was taking glucophage.

Here was the living proof of my thesis that a non-diabetic could be a diabetic. The critical action was the doctor identifying Dave as a diabetic. He must have recognized the difference between a hypoglycemian and a hyperglycemian. He probably saved Dave from neuropathy, macular degeneration, and the other serious complication of diabetes.

I had a copy of my book with me, and gave it to Dave. I suggested to Dave to continue the medicine, but follow the supplements and diets recommended in the book. As he saw his glucose number progress downward towards 70, start to decrease the medication until he could be consistently under the critical reading. From time to time, inform the doctor of his progress. Also, ask his doctor to conduct an analysis to see if there would be any adverse reaction between the medicine and the supplements. I will have to meet his doctor! What a gem.

## *Others*

Recently I had an opportunity to talk with John B., a friend from New Hampshire.

"I have changed my diet and am feeling great," he said. "I appreciate the advice on foods you gave me when last we chatted."

John still looked about 20 or so pounds overweight.

"What is your number?" I asked.

"Its okay."

"What can you remember of the number?"

"Ah, it was 91 and that's very good."

"No, John, that's very bad."

"Well 91 is certainly within a range of 70 to 120 isn't it? The doctor said it was at my last checkup."

Of all the hyper's I have talked with, none have ever said that they got below 98. Therefore, a 91 must be a hypo. I explained this to John, and indicated that he was 21 points above his safe glucose number. I gave him a copy of my book.

## Helping Our Wounded

When a diabetic has already developed some of the serious complications of diabetes, they need help. This help should begin with everyone helping them to develop the desire, to slow down the progression of the complication. Don't just live with it as it becomes worse, without trying to stop it from getting worse.

Changing one's lifestyle, the right diet, taking supplements, use of the mind, is basic to reaching this goal. In addition, there may be technological advances that could help lessen the problem of the serious complication of the disease.


## Neuropathy

For those with neuropathy, our wounded friends, the first fighting approach is to stop eating the things that cause it. You need to slow down, to zero, if possible, the progression of the disease. Those with neuropathy need to follow the diet and supplement recommendations, and other additions to the program.

I have yet to hear the medical community say with a consistent voice, what causes neuropathy. I also have met those with fairly serious cases say they don't know what causes it, but it's not diabetes. These are the ones with a glucose reading of 85 to 90. Hypoglycemians?

Who cares if you believe that you are not a diabetic? Why not jump in one's canoe that seems to be reaching safety, by practicing what this book teaches, whatever you call, or don't call one's self?

A standard current medical approach is to prescribe medicine. Unfortunately, this is not to rid oneself of neuropathy, or even slow down its progression towards gangrene. It is meant to lessen the pain. The job of this painkiller is to deaden the transmitters of the damaged nerves, so that the brain doesn't get the pain signals. The dosage of the medicine is increased over time as the pain increases, or the neuropathy continues to progress from feet, to leg, to thigh. This is where we are in the treatment of neuropathy. A commonly prescribed medicine is amitriptylin in ten mg tablets. This is a substitute for Elavil. These drugs are traditionally prescribed as antidepressants. They, in this case, apparently treat the damaged nerve endings, and the transmission of pain to the brain.

If we are following a self-help approach, we need to get help for the "wounds." If it is possible to provide some better circulation, without the person just using the painkiller to keep the situation somewhat muted, then it should be seen as worth trying to do something about it.

### *Foot and Leg Massages*

I discovered foot and leg massage equipments in a catalog on a plane ride from the West to the East coast. The name of the company that produces these units is Footsmart. They advertise smarter, better products for lower body health. They are out of Norcross, GA and are probably not the only company that produces similar products.

I liked the words in their advertisement for air compression boots, and air compression legs – "Sequential compression therapy enhances leg circulation." This company also advertises, "walk-care" – reduces pain and enhances the blood flow. A friend of mine is trying the leg and boot compression units. She says that they make her feet and legs "feel better." Interesting in that her neurologist told her a while back that she essentially does not have any feeling in her feet.

Time will tell on what benefits it will provide. But it's probably better than doing nothing. She is a fighter, and trying to use every weapon she can to restore her walking ability. This equipment costs over $200 and may be out of the reach of many individuals. But this is what family and friends are for.

If this equipment can stimulate the nerves to increase circulation, it would be a big asset in containing or eliminating neuropathy.  If not, there is at least hope in that there are companies working on more technique development that can provide better circulation in the future.

### *Oxygen Therapy*

GWR Medical Inc. claims to be the first in topical hyper baric oxygen therapy.  They can be seen on www.thbo.com.  Their brochure is very graphic.  One of their examples shows a 71-year-old male diabetic with a full thickness wound on his forefoot.  Amputation of the entire foot was recommended after three months of non-healing.  THBO Therapy healed the wound completely in 84 days.

## _Macular Degeneration_

The macular is the central part of the retina, and contains the area needed for all central and fine vision. The medical community says that for reasons unknown, yellowish deposits (drusen) form in the macular, which tends to damage the retina and create a loss of vision. For what we have learned so far, I make the assumption that the yellowish deposits are caused by the glucose, particularly when some have transformed into free radicals. We know that macular degeneration is a serious consequence of diabetes, and until proven wrong, we can assume that most, if not all, macular degeneration is caused by diabetes.

Let's see what we know, or can theorize, to help this group of our wounded. Let's see what else the medical community knows as reported in the _"Health Care Network"_. They state "Macular degeneration, for the most part, is age related to people over the age of fifty. It is associated with a family history".

Here we go again. People eating the wrong stuff over a long period of time ("age related') will get diabetes, and therefore will develop some of its serious consequences. If most of the family is eating the same wrong stuff ("family history"), then they will all probably get diabetes.

_Health Care Network_ goes on to say, "The disease is not well understood as to its risk factors and etiology." Isn't that the same as saying that the medical community doesn't have a clue? Etiology is medicalease for saying, the assignment of cause, origin or reason for something.

_Health Care Network_ further says, "Our treatment of the disease is very lacking. The only proven treatment is with a laser and only for the wet form of the disease. Laser treatment may be an option to prevent deterioration of the vision. In many cases in which laser is performed, the vision can continue to deteriorate." This means that this laser treatment is very risky. However, some will go for it because they don't want to face the progression to blindness.

If the person continues to eat or drink the stuff that started the vision deterioration in the first place, then it would be expected that the laser is only correcting the condition at that time. Further damage will occur by continuing to ingest the wrong stuff. The answer, we now know, is in going to the right diet, developing fighters by taking the right supplements, and mellowing out.

It is interesting to see an article in the *"New York Times"*, since I wrote these words. A study by the National Eye Institute of more than 3,600 patients showed that high doses of antioxidants and the mineral zinc could reduce the progression of diabetes by about 25%. Dr. Thomas Friberg of the Eye and Ear Institute (NEI) at the University of Pittsburgh said there was no previous therapy to prevent the progression of macular degeneration.

This continues to point out the difficulties that our American medical community has had treating complications of diabetes sufficiently. But progress is being made.

The NEI study report does not identify the antioxidants, or their dosages. Of significant importance to the diabetic, the report does not identify the source of the macular degeneration, which we know could be our enemy, diabetes. This investigation is significant, and is on the right track, and it would be encouraging if they continue to look at all of the supplements, and identify the cause of the macular degeneration.

Patients with macular degeneration are treated by careful monitoring of the patient about every three months. There are two aspects of this monitoring. One is a measure of vision – the ability to see. There will be a gradual deterioration of the distance, and clarity of what can be seen. The remedy, eyeglasses that "correct" the problem, as it increases.

The second aspect of monitoring is the perceived health of the eye. The ophthalmologist looks behind the eye for various conditions, such as bleeding, and even to view warts. There are medical treatments for these conditions.

There are two hopes to slow the progression and hopefully to bring it to a halt. One is to <u>stop ingesting the wrong stuff.</u> The second is to take supplements in the recommended dosages, no more, no less. Take the recommended program. Vitamin E is highly recommended as we have already discussed. Be sure to take B-6 because it enhances Vitamin E. Be sure to take zinc too. Try bilberry as well. You want fighters that can fight the free radicals that are attacking your eyes. Remember that the blood carriers in your eyes, the capillaries, are very small, and objects such as glucose can become more significant in the small diameters of the capillaries.

Look for <u>respected</u> medical reports that have clear, documented information that are useful for macular degeneration.

One such report is from Dr. David Williams, the author of "Alternatives".[6] In the dry form of macular degeneration, the tiny blood vessels feeding the macular are essentially starved of oxygen and nutrients, because the capillaries are clogged.

A <u>promising</u> new treatment option is to use very small electric currents to stimulate blood flow to the eye. This is the approach of Dr. Merrill Allen of the Indiana University of Optometry. The stimulator operates on 9 volts with an output of 200 microamperes at 10 cycles per second. This stimulation process improved blood flow to the eye and appeared to trigger regrowth of the retina, and photoreceptors in the eye.

---

[6] Alternatives, Mountain Home Publishing, PO Box 61010 Rockville MD 20859

A group of Dr. Allen's patients gained an amazing average of 8.5 letters of acuity per eye on the eye chart.

More research results are needed to prove the benefits of this technique. The process looks valid enough to warrant our close scrutiny. Also, there is a need to develop an inexpensive test unit, and a simple test procedure in order to make this potential eye-saver serve the needs of many people.

Those that practice The Silva Method will recognize the parameter 10 cycles per second as a healing frequency. Perhaps one of their leaders could visualize a small audio transmitter, like a small tape recorder. This recorder would have just the 10 cycles per second sound on it. The recorder would be held close to the eye. It would cause a vibration in the physical portions of the eye. This may induce the type of healing similar to Dr. Allen's.

There are many paths to healing.

## *Specific Supplements and Diet*

In general, we know that diet and supplements as described in this book, should be able to help our wounded. Let's be specific. The nine recommended supplements for macular degeneration include eight that we have already recommended. They are beta-carotene, bilberry, grape seed extract, selenium, Vitamin A, Vitamin C, Vitamin E, and zinc. The ninth is shark cartilage, which is taken to prevent, and possibly halt, the progression of the wet form of macular degeneration.

As for diet, eat plenty of blueberries, blackberries, and cherries. Also, raw fruits and vegetables. Follow the GI index for the best carbohydrates to avoid helping the enemy.

By fighting against diabetes, we are trying to avoid getting to the stages of the complications of the diseases of our wounded. But, those with the head start on having diabetes are our brothers and sisters too. Perhaps some of this information can help. I am sure there is other information useful for the other serious complication of diabetes. If so, let's get this information out of there into everyone's hands that need it. Major health organizations in the United States and abroad, major talk show hosts, our government leaders and so on, can help.

## Susceptibility Because of Diabetes

An acquaintance of mine told me his doctor wanted to amputate his leg in two weeks. He believed that it was because he was a diabetic that he was to have this harrowing experience. He rationalized that because he is a diabetic, that other "attacks" on his body that usually would cause a normal reaction, became a very serious threat to his health. If he went ahead and gave into an operation, it would mean a drastic change in his lifestyle.

This is his story, as told in his words. His name is Waldo, and he is a senior construction engineer.

"In the summer of 1999, I was constructing a new road in a nearby town. During construction, I scrapped my leg about 4 inches above the ankle on bull briers, the worst kind. It didn't seem to be more than a scratch. After a few weeks, it didn't seem to heal and I realized that it must be an ulcerated wound, due to my having diabetes." (*Author's note* – "an ulcerated wound is defined as an inflammatory, often suppurating (to form, or discharge pus) lesion, resulting in an internal mucous surface of the body, resulting in necrosis of the tissue".)

"I then went to a local diabetic clinic and proceeded to use the medicines and solutions that they recommended. I would go at least once a week. After approximately one year, there were no results, and the injury was getting deeper and larger. I was informed that surgery might be the only cure."

"At this point I was not too happy with the expert. I left the clinic and went home, upset and wondering what to do with myself. I felt my world had left me. What now?"

"I picked up the yellow pages and started going through it, looking for some specialist in that field. After about five yellow page books, I picked up the book of a town about 15 miles away. I found Dr. K. listed. He is a diabetic injury specialist. I called him and explained my worsening problem. As it was about 5pm, I thought that he would want me to make an appointment as soon as possible. He surprised me. He asked how long it would take me to get to his office. I replied, about 20 minutes, and he said he would wait."

"As I drove, I thought, what can he do that the clinic couldn't in a year? My "scratch" was now the size of a silver dollar and right down to the bone! I really had no hope and thought that I would lose my leg to diabetes."

"The second I arrived at his office, Dr. K. was at the door waiting for me." "Come right in, hop up on the examining table and let me take a look."

"Mmmmm", he said. "Looks like <u>we</u> have a problem, but I think I can help you." "After explaining everything from the injury and the clinic, the care, meals, etc., Dr. K. asked me about medicines and solutions." "Wrong, wrong, wrong. Do not use those anymore."

At that point, he asked if I liked tea and I said no. He then proceeded to remove some dead tissue around my injury and then disappeared. When he came back, he had a cup of tea. He explained that chamomile tea is a healing tea. Yeah, and the moon is made of cheese! He asked me to drink a cup of tea with him, and I said sure, why not. We then sat, and drank the tea. Dr. K. then took the hot tea bag and applied it to the wound! After ten minutes, the bag was cool and he removed it, and then sprinkled polysporin powder on it and then the good doctor disappeared again, only to return with hot cabbage leaves, which he wrapped around the injury and secured it with gauze and tape. At that point, Dr. K. said he wanted to see me tomorrow, same time! I continued to visit the doctor every day for approximately one and a half weeks. We noticed that junny (like spider web) crossing the bone." The doctor said, "Flesh is starting to grow." "At that time, I would visit every 3 days. Three weeks later, he did the same process but left the cabbage leaves off and added a magnet directly over the wound and taped it there. I also added magnetic soles to my shoes, which made my feet feel much better. He advised me that magnets help open the capillaries to increase blood flow.

A few weeks went by and I noticed the injury was getting shallower and smaller. At that point, I began seeing Dr. K. once a month. He informed me to change my diet because being a type O positive blood type eating carbohydrates, is really putting poison into my system. He told me to eat more green vegetables and fresh fruit. He also said no ham, although I could eat red meat. I was to limit my consumption of eggs to three a week. He also said drink lots of fluids. It has been four years now and I feel fine, with the advice of Dr. K. and the meals he recommended have brought my diabetic level down from 250 plus, to a pretty steady 118. My injury is gone completely with the exception of some discoloration! The good doctor explained to me that the color is the last thing to change and may never return to normal skin color.

I believe that Dr. K. has saved my life and I owe it to him. I firmly believe that there are alternate treatments for healing and it all starts with blood type and eating the right foods.

What are the important things in Waldo's story? Waldo went looking through the yellow pages. He took responsibility for his health! He recognized that any "attacks" to his diabetic body could encounter a reduced immune system fighting off diabetes. Therefore, he needed special treatment. Doctors should be sensitive to susceptibility concerns for diabetics experiencing other medical problems. Interesting that diet played a role, and magnets can be helpful healers. Dr. K. believes that blood type also plays a role. You may want to look at Dr. Peter J.D. Adamo's book on this subject (reading list). There is incentive in ridding our bodies of diabetes as soon as possible, before it makes us vulnerable to other medical problems.

Dr. K. is a European doctor. If interested, and if Waldo agrees, information on Waldo and Dr. K. can be provided by contacting the author at the publisher.

"The power of people doing things for themselves is very strong medicine."

Kate Loring,  R.N.  Dr.  P.H. Director of Patient Education

Stanford Arthritis Center, Professor School of Medicine

## *Program Summary*

We have been on an interesting journey together.  We now have information that we have discovered that could change our lives forever.

We didn't know what diabetes was.  My first way of explaining it to others was to say that it is a condition of the body when my glucose reading was too high.  I now know <u>what</u> diabetes is. It is free radicals that have resulted from glucose changing its form, due to oxidation.  Then these free radicals attack my body.  Something like a butterfly emerging from a "worm".  Friends who have arthritis can only tell me their symptoms, not the cause.

Ok, you have diabetes!  Or a family member, or friend, has diabetes.  You must take on the fight yourself to get rid of it, or help others to rid themselves of it.

You now know what causes it.  More importantly, who causes it – you.

<u>What you should do</u> –

- change your diet
- start monitoring your glucose number
- adjust your living habits, if necessary, to stay on your program
- start taking the recommended supplements
- practice stress reduction
- use the additional programs to enhance your program

<u>What you should do for others</u> –

- tell others of your accomplishments
- encourage them to have a physical, or at least, take the finger-prick test
- tell them to get their own copy of this self-help book, for ridding themselves of diabetes, or to use it as a diabetic prevention aid
- explain to others that they may be non-diabetic that is a diabetic

We as "doctors", have to make decisions as to advising the patient, us, what to do about any long-term trend. This includes the concern of potential deterioration of our body when at diabetic's levels. These decisions can include getting serious about following a program for better health, like Fighting Diabetes.

There are diet concepts that can work for you to help avoid the potential severe complications of diabetes.

Adjust your living style where necessary. Leave room in your living for very occasional deviations from your program. Monitor closely the lasting affect on your blood sugar. You will need to make healthy changes to your lifestyle. You will need to stay motivated to help you achieve your goals. One of the better ways is to tell others of your plan to change.

Take the recommended supplements daily and at the correct dosage. Some provide the fighters to stop the enemy free radicals you created, from attacking your body tissues. Others, like the trace minerals, replace missing items in our foods. We also take supplements as helpers in insulin production and in utilization by the cells. This is important when the pump has difficulty producing sufficient insulin.

Reduce the amount of stress you accept in your life, through the way you interpret events happening to you. The three most useful words, spoken or unspoken, between two people, may not be "I Love You", but "Let It Be". When used, doesn't "Let It Be" tend to diffuse a negative situation, when essentially the other person may not really understand the negative impact that they are creating? Could it end up being a benefit to both parties? Who needs negative juices circulating in their bodies?

Practice affirmations by building on Emil Coue's "day-by-day in every way, I am getting better and better". You can invent a particular diabetic affirmation, such as "I desire that my body and subconscious mind eliminate diabetes from me". Concentrate on being thankful for what you have, and less on what you don't have. Use your mind and see how to develop a mind-body link.

Exercise is helpful, to all of us, in varying degrees of helping. Exercise is the user of fuel in the cells that were stored there by the conversion of glucose into fuel. That allows glucose still in the bloodstream to come into the cells. This helps. But if we continue to create excess fuel (glucose) in our bloodstream, by eating the wrong foods, all the exercise we can normally do will not be able to handle all of the excess fuel.

For exercise to be effective, dedicate yourself to some scheduled time to do the exercise(s) you like. If you say you can't find the time, you are only saying you didn't give it a higher priority. We all get 24 hours a day, 7 days a week. It is reported that those who have lived a life of hard physical activity, tend to live longer. Be one of them.

Small changes in lifestyle can help. Chewing, cooking, sufficient water, avoiding saturated fats, all can help.

Say to yourself, I am in charge of my body's health. Occasionally, I will need some professional help, but I am the one on a day-to-day basis that must practice my self-help program.

For the non-insulin dependent diabetic, getting rid of diabetes is really quite simple. No, there is no "magic bullet". You don't need one. Dedicated, persistent effort to be sure, but no quick fix.

An old saying, "the program works if you work the program". It is amazingly true. When we see our glucose suddenly high, it is usually when we are off the program, are under tremendous stress, or our immune system is fighting another problem. Once we understand the cause, we can initiate corrective action, before it is too late. If we can reason out that our immune system is heavily occupied in fighting another attack on our immune system, don't worry about your number. Just say, 'body, thank you for fighting off this other threat'.

Don't expect to win the fight against diabetes in a very short time. This is not a magic bullet approach. Open your mouth and take this magic potion and you instantly win the battle. It took you awhile, at least months if not years, doing the wrong things to get it, and it will now take a reasonable time, although much shorter time, to overcome this debilitating killer. My experience was that it took about 7 months to get to the 103-105 glucose levels from a 168 number.

Included in that time period were learning, testing, and developing the program. Your time period should be appreciably less.

If we have diabetes, to get rid of it, we will have to change. We have caused it! People want to do things the same way that they have been doing them. They often feel change is fearful, or at least unpleasant.

The clue is to visualize ourselves after we change. There should be no fear of the serious complication, or early death, no fear of the path ahead. The ability to be there for our children, our loved ones. The missed opportunities to be you.

Helping Others – Help the people who are unknowingly heading toward amputation, blindness, or other diabetic complications, because they are naturally hypoglycemias, and their high glucose reading is masked by being evaluated within a range, instead of a difference from their natural healthy state.

Try to help children, yours, your grandchildren, and children of friends. As any "teacher", you may have trouble succeeding, but the effort is worth it if you save a child from this silent killer.

Follow The Basic 60-Day Program. Set goals for yourself. Paraphrasing Alice in Wonderland, "if you don't know where you are going, than any road will get you there."

A Harvard University study of their graduates determined the more successful had goals. The most successful, wrote them down. You will need some discipline, in being goal oriented. You can do it. Walk the walk and talk the talk. Some will be listening when they understand what you are achieving, and will want your success.

Be the best you can be and the best you can be for others.

## *The Basic 60-Day Program*

Weeks 1 and 2


Start Slow Digestion Diet

Eliminate white –
  Rice
  Potatoes
  Flour Products

And eliminate
  Dried fruits
  Parsnip
  Tofu, frozen dessert
  Tapioca Pudding
  Jelly Beans

Take Essential Supplements (Masison Modified Supplement List) –
  Drink 6 oz. of water first; take supplements with remaining 6 oz.
  L-Carnitine        take 500 twice a day
  L-Glutamine        take 500 twice a day
  Taurine            take 500 twice a day
  Alpha Lipoic       take 300 twice a day
  Chromium
  Zinc
  Biotin

The Self-Test Program –
  Record what you eat & drink
  Test your glucose reading
  Before your first meal, take your reading, Mon-Fri
  Record your reading
  Review yesterdays eating, drinking

Next Day, Repeat Steps Again
  Analyze changes in your reading from yesterday
  Determine if some food or drink my be increasing your level
  If so, modify your eating habits

Develop Stress Reduction Techniques
  During the day, find opportunities to say, "Day by Day, I am getting Better and Better"
  Practice reducing the time spent in a negative mood, angry, frustrated, disappointed, etc.

Weeks 3 and 4


Continue Program from weeks 1 and 2

Eliminate Some Foods
        Corn & corn products, except popcorn
        Carefully select breakfast cereals
                Best – oatmeal
                Worst – cereals with much sugar, like frosty, glazed, honey
        Eliminate flour products such as donuts, pretzels, most cookies & cakes
        Pumpkin and watermelon

Reduce the amount of colas in your diet

Start the Reduced Carbo diet
        Add eggs, meat, fish, and chicken to replace some carbs

Don't eat foods with hydrogenated additives

Add "very important" supplements
        C-Q-10
        Magnesium
        Manganese
        Also folic and B-12 together, and vitamins A-C-E
                A is in the form of Beta Carotene
        B-6 to strengthen Vitamin E

Continue using the Self-Test Program
        Use your meter's data storage capability
        Check your 30-day average
        If reasonably lower than when you started, celebrate!
        If the same, or higher, contact me at the publishers

Continue Stress Reduction Techniques

Incorporate "Let it be" into your thinking
        Prepare and then practice this, when negative emotions start to flow

Take at least 15 minutes a day to do nothing
        Settle your mind and rid yourself of mental muck

<u>Weeks 5 and 6</u>


<u>Continue Program from weeks 3 and 4</u>

<u>Get omega 3's into your diet</u>
>Fresh water fish –
>>Alaska/wild Salmon
>>Swordfish
>>Haddock, Cod, Mackerel
>>Other sources –
>>>Add flaxseeds and walnuts to your foods
>>>Flaxseeds have a higher concentration of omega 3's than salmon
>>>The seeds are more beneficial than the oil

<u>Add Important Supplements</u>
>Selenium, Potassium
>Bilberry, Pyconogenol
>Coral Calcium

<u>Continue Using the Self-Test Program</u>
>If you have been taking insulin, and your glucose reading
>>is going down, tell your doctor and see if he wants to initiate
>>a reduced insulin program.

<u>Incorporate more stress reduction techniques</u>
>Continue the practice of balancing your life with small periods of mental relaxation
>Tapes help, and there are many good sources

<u>New Uses for your Mind</u>
>Learn simple relaxation techniques. Try to find some time
>>to incorporate meditation into your schedule
>Discover how to meditate and try the techniques of
>>visualization and imagination; often just before
>>going to sleep helps

<u>Social Support</u>
>Enlist the support of your spouse and family in your program
>>and in its success. They can help you, and you may be
>>able to help them.
>Don't insist on your loved ones joining you in doing what you are doing,
>>but educate them on what you are doing, and ask for their support.

Weeks 7 and 8

Continue  Program from weeks 6 and 7

Supplements
      You could add gymnema and fenugreek to your
          supplement program.  Your fundamental program
          should be enough, but they could provide some help.
      Read the "Glucose Revolution" for further review of foods
          that you like to eat but are not listed in this book.

Continue Using the Self-Test Program
      Become aware of finger prick testing techniques
          available in your pharmacy.
      Throw away your old calendars on which you recorded
          consumed food/beverages, and your glucose readings.
      They have done their job in helping you to develop the
          discipline that you needed to be on a daily program of
          improvement.

Adjust your living habits
      You, too, can eat a cheeseburger with only using one of
          the buns, or a wrap.
      Relish your role as the day-to-day doctor.  You will be
          seeing the data that the doctor could not reasonably be expected
          to see.  You can take day-to-day action to help your health.
      Reduce the amount of stress you accept in your life, through the
          ways you interpret events happening to you.

      Even though exercise may be only a 10% factor in ridding oneself of diabetes, you may
          want to have an exercise program.  After all, when you are at a glucose reading of
          120, 10% will bring you to 108.  Exercise can exist on its own merits in helping
          your body to be in general good health.

Just repeat these 8 weeks (60 days) over and over, and rid yourself of diabetes.

## *Epilogue*

I participated in many sports going through school. I was the captain of several teams. Later in life, I was always competitive. This was whether in my career, when I founded several companies and competed in the marketplace, or in a simple game of cards.

Fighting off diabetes was at first a game. I needed my best effort and a desire to win. The objective was to lower the glucose reading. There were many trial and error approaches. There were small victories and a few large ones.

Then the realization came, it was no longer a game of numbers. It was a game of life! I realized that it was not just the pursuit of a lower number each day, or week. With a number higher than 110-120, I was doing damage to my body each day! I was heading for <u>those severe</u> <u>complications</u>, putting my heart, eyes, kidney, limbs, etc. in danger. This was no game; to do your best, it was a fight for a normal life. Forget how I got there, it is now a fight that I must win. The first step was a critical analysis of what in my lifestyle could be contributing to my having a disease.

Along the way, I learned that this game of life had more truths than I had imagined. I was changing my lifestyle. I was not just popping supplements, or experimenting with diets. In a practical sense, I had to learn to be different than many others. I had to refrain from certain fast-digestion foods, to not eat peanuts or snacks at night, to tell a waitress I did not wish to choose among baked, mashed, red bliss potatoes, or rice to go with my entrée. I asked for a double order of vegetables, or found something in the listing of side dishes. I had to go from a sandwich, to trying to eat a sandwich with only one slice of bread. I had to translate what I had read about – the glycemic index – into the practical practice of my life.

There were social adjustments as well as culinary. There were many more changes I had to put into practice as I learned more about what in my lifestyle was contributing to my having diabetes. I had to really probe and understand stress reduction. I had to evaluate, for my use, affirmations, mediation, etc. There were affirmations that I believed were useful. I made them up. I had to try to trace back and identify cause and affect relationships. What were the real sources of stress? I tried to shift some of my activities.

I came to realize there were some fundamental truths of interrelationships that many of us learned, but never practice. Remember in the Lord's Prayer when you say, "forgive us our trespasses, <u>as</u> we forgive those who trespass against us." Sounds simple enough as we remember the first part. Do we expect forgiveness whether we forgive or not? It's a very big step to go beyond practicing forgiveness. Thinking of giving someone a little slack is only a beginning. To truly extend the hand of friendship to all who come into our life is more demanding of us. It takes a shift in our value systems. But it can go a long way to reducing stress in your life as well as becoming a positive force in your relationships. I'm not saying that I have achieved substantial gains in this aspect of life, but I am aware, and am working on it. It will be the same for anyone, as you realize you truly do have control over your life, and can virtually be anything you want to be. You can rid yourself of the dangers of diabetes, and probably most other health problems. Seek out knowledge. The lack of it is killing us. There is a lot that is not very useful. However, you will find gems that can help you if you have the mindset that they should come to you. Use the information to your benefit. Take time to reflect on yourself, who you are, where you are going in life, what happened to your dreams, what happened to your relationships.

Be kind to yourself. Enjoy your life. You are only issued one.

As a motivation to you, as I write these words, I can report to you that my glucose reading this morning was 98, 70 points below my high point. I won the fight! Now you go ahead and win yours.

## _What if?_

Just think about it.  Without diabetic patients arriving at doctor's offices, clinics, hospitals, university medical centers, government and commercial facilities, for –

1 – Doctors and nurses providing periodic checkups using glucose readings,

2 – Doctors renewing prescriptions and pharmacies filling them,

3 – Nurse, under the supervision of doctors washing diabetic patients' kidneys, each three times a week, with the aid of expensive dialysis machines,

4 – Ophthalmologists conducting eye exams to see how the eye's macular degeneration is progressing, providing treatment for bleeding, and upgrading eye glass prescriptions,

5 – Neurologists observing the progression of loss of feeling in limbs, of patients, as neuropathy progresses from toes to ankles to knees, increasing the dosages of painkillers, and eventually scheduling amputation,

6 – Cardiologists and nurses conducting blood tests, EGG, various scan techniques, and other tests to determine changes in heart performance leading to possible heart failure, and

7 – Frustrated administrators telling veterans there are no beds that are available for them to receive treatment, for lack of resources, doctors, nurses, and facilities.

There could be –

1 – University, government, and commercial research labs re-directing their resources to fight other health problems,

2 – Insurance companies able to shift from payments of benefits to its diabetic customers, to focus on better management of resources for revenue enhancement, and provide better insurance products at affordable prices,

3 – Further think and see all of the above seven resources being applied to other health fighting needs, such as –

    1 – Fighting arthritis
    2- Fighting asthma
    3- Fighting alzheimer's
    4- Fighting heart disease
    5- Fighting cancer

And of course, the list goes on. Wouldn't it be great if we could put adult diabetes behind us, along with obesity, and focus valuable resources on other major killers at work around the world?

Millions of dollars now being used less effectively could be applied to the juvenile diabetic eradication, additional treatment centers for the wounded with the severe complication of diabetes, and education programs for diabetic prevention, and to convert less wounded diabetics to recovering diabetics. Government agencies, pharmaceutical research labs and many other activities would still have roles to perform, but the focus would change.

There are members of Congress getting ready to propose additional hundreds of millions of dollars to be spent on diabetes to find the "magic bullet" in some unknown research lab somewhere. A refocus is needed. This new focus would use savings from the current and proposed additional millions to look at other diseases that may be a threat to us because of a lack of good nutritional knowledge. These might include arthritis, heart disease and cancer.

Enough people utilizing the Fighting Diabetes Program, as successfully as the author, would mean that some of the saved millions now used in diabetic treatment programs, can go to the homeless, in this and other countries, the underprivileged, the uneducated, the less fortunate here and abroad, that could help in turning their lives around, and contribute to the quality of life in America, and in the world.

## *Appendix*

Our knowledge of diabetes and general health keeps changing like an elusive enemy, and also our counterattack capability changes too using the results of on-going research. New approaches to some items can be added to our self-help approach.

Some approaches can provide possible <u>changes</u> to what we already know. Some will be <u>additions</u> to what we know, and some will address what we can do to <u>help</u> those with serious complications of diabetes. All of these will represent a section of the book that should continue to expand and enlighten the reader.

Whether <u>changes,</u> <u>additions,</u> or <u>help</u>; more <u>Fighting Diabetes</u> research may be needed to provide us the opportunity to analyze whether they should be part of our basic program. Our self-help goal remains to rid ourselves of diabetes.


## *General Health*

There are many things that we can do for our general health. If they give us a stronger immune system to fight off illnesses and diseases, than that is of interest to us as we fight diabetes.

On the other hand, if they give diseases the upper hand, by weakening our immune system, then we are interested in that too. We will look at some food items to illustrate this point.

If it can be said that we have a strong immune system, there is a belief among a certain minority of the American medical community that will say that your body can ward off everything from a cold to a cancer. There may be some validity for this point of view. Whether we accept this point of view, we have come this far, to know to ask; show me the evidence. And there may be <u>some</u>. From our viewpoint, it is clear that we do not want to be at a disadvantage in our fight against diabetes. If other things are occurring that could weaken our bodies, it's like putting out a fire in our living quarters, and then discovering that the roof is on fire.

There is significant evidence to be able to say that smoking can cause serious problems, if continued in excess, over a number of years. The same case can be said for a severe case of alcoholism. Doctors are now saying, those with diabetes, should be very moderate drinkers.

In addition to my detailed diabetes research, I began to add areas of general health to investigate. My reasoning is that even if we solve the diabetes problem, there still could be a total body problem that could diminish our hard fought victory over diabetes.

My assumption here is that we are fighting one problem, diabetes that our body needs to prevent, or get rid of, within a body that is not in a survival status, due to other self-inflicted wounds.

Going forward with this assumption, let's see if some common food items can strengthen or weaken our immune system.

| __Food Item__ | __Strengthen or Weaken?__ |
|---|---|
| Salmon | Maybe yes or no |
| Cinnamon | Strengthen |
| Vinegar | Strengthen |
| Popcorn | Surprisingly OK |
| Coffee | Strengthen |
| Chocolate | OK, at least for males |

## Salmon

Natural salmon is an excellent food. Among its benefits is the omega 3 it contains. There is now a question of farmed salmon, where the salmon is put into pens on land and essentially farmed fed and harvested. The *Health Bytes Newsletter* reported that an "Environmental Working Group" (EWG), bought and tested farmed salmon filets from ten grocery stores in Washington, Oregon, and California. They found seven stores contained high levels of Polychlorinated Biphenysis (PCB). With 52 million Americans eating salmon, thus creating a very large demand for salmon, this can be a very serious threat to the nations' health.

There is a report from *Bottom Line Health* that points out that farmed salmon are fattened with soybean pellets, dosed with antibiotics, and injected with synthetic dye that gives them their pink color. This, at first thought, may not seem to be too harmful to us. The report goes on to say that farmed salmon contain 2/3rds less omega 3. They also cite the PCB's.

PCB's, have been identified as a cancer causing danger. Other reports on salmon indicate that the pellets the salmon are fed contain other ingredients that are not healthy for us.

There needs to be immediate testing of farmed salmon to discern the potential danger to us. Perhaps the FDA is a likely agency to study this potential problem, and if appropriate, issue health warnings, and find a way to invoke remedial actions. This not only applies to the techniques of farming, but also to labeling. Only trust, at this time, Alaska and Wild labeled salmon.

Many of our nutritional gurus have advocated eating salmon twice a week to obtain their normally large amounts of omega 3s. We seem to get enough omega 6s in our normal diet. The 3s are needed to create a healthy balance of omegas for our bodies.

## Cinnamon

A new book, "Eat and Heal" by Gayle K. Ward, is coming out shortly. In it, Gayle makes a case for the use of cinnamon to lower blood sugar. She says sprinkling as little as 1/8<sup>th</sup> of a teaspoon on a dessert, applesauce, putting it in tea, or on toast, "can triple the body's ability to metabolize blood sugar."

It sounds like it makes sense and it is nice to have another fighter on our side, but it needs empirical verification. The same procedure should be followed, try it and measure the results. Of course, in addition to us converts practicing self-help, it would be nice to have some research labs also testing cinnamon.

## Vinegar

I have recently learned that vinegar is good for you. Vinegar contains acids, which delay stomach emptying. This slows down digestion in the small intestine. This gives the pancreas the opportunity to produce, and send forth the needed insulin. I have gone to raspberry vinaigrette for my salad dressing.

## Popcorn

For the sharp reader, you will have picked up the difference in the GI ratings between corn and popcorn. In the low GI foods listing, popcorn has a rating of only 55 compared to corn with a high GI rating of 75-84.

This favorite for carnivals, movies, ballgame goers, and backyard parties, has the corn kernels undergoing changes to its very structure when heated during cooking (popping) that then causes a lower, and more desirable GI value.

## *Coffee*

I was surprised to learn that Dr. Willard Willet, renown Harvard Nutritionist does not try to avoid coffee and go to tea. He believes "coffee in moderation is benign, even beneficial." Too much can be a problem. Coffee drinkers have fewer kidney stones and gallstones.

## *Chocolate*

Quite a few medical reports are now advocating eating chocolate. Penney-Kris Etherton, PhD, RD, distinguished Professor of Nutrition at Penn State University, has found that people who ate a diet rich in cocoa powder, and dark chocolate, had lower oxidation levels of bad LDL cholesterol, higher blood antioxidant levels, and 4% higher levels of good cholesterol. Dr. Kris-Etherton states, "research shows that a diet containing about an ounce of chocolate a day increases good cholesterol and prevents bad cholesterol from oxidizing, a process that may lead to heart disease.

It appears that the chocolate with highest cocoa content (dark chocolate) has the highest flavanol content and therefore is best for you.

*Bottom Line Newsletter* has a report from the *British Medical Journal* that identifies chocolate as having a remarkable longevity benefit for men. All it takes is just a "few pieces of chocolate a month for men to live significantly longer. Researchers believe the antioxidant compounds in chocolate, similar to those found in red wine, are the main reason for longevity."

*Prevention* magazine's February issue, way back in 2003, said much the same.

They quantified it by saying "Just one ounce packs more than twice the healthy antioxidant punch of red wine." They qualified it to a particular dark chocolate, Dove Dark. This chocolate, made by Mars, contains a specially processed cocoa. Harold Schmitz, director of science at Mars states that studies show lower risk of heart disease, lung cancer, prostate cancer, asthma, and type 2 diabetes.

Chocoholics of the world unite!

## _Supplements Further Research_

Supplements are sold at the GNC, Vitamin World, and other health stores, as well at drug stores and food stores. You can buy them through the mail or on the Internet. Packaging, cost, quality, can vary. It comes down to convenience of shopping, price, available dosages, and your perception of quality. Perception will depend on your understanding as to how these factors work for you. Remember, you are the day-to-day doctor.

Further information research appearing since I have almost completed this book, is some recommended changes to the supplements. We must judge these new items carefully, making sure that the information is not premature, without a complete evaluation of their potential capabilities and possible side-affects.

We will look at –

Potential changes to the Balch Recommendations

Availability of supplements

Chromium Polynicotinate

Folic Acid – New Form, Folinate

And a Masison Modified Supplement List

I never found Quercetin in the supplement stores I shopped. I found that food served me well here.

I only found Biotin as 600 mcg, not 50mg, and I take the 600 mcg, which is less than 1 mg.

I only found Inositol as 500 mg, rather than 50 mg, and I do not take the 500.

I found magnesium at 500 mg, rather than 750, and that works for me.

I found Bilberry at 60 mg, and I take it.

I changed Vitamin A to Beta Carotene.  I found out that too much Vitamin A is not good for us.  Remember, you get some Vitamin A from the food you eat, as well as taking a supplement. Beta Carotene is like a pre-vitamin A, in that our bodies change the beta-carotene into Vitamin A.  The good news is that our smart bodies do not make the change unless our bodies really need more Vitamin A.  Excess beta-carotene will be used as energy, or simply passed on through our bodies.

These changes continued to help me rid myself of diabetes.  By the way, I have written Dr. James Balch several times, to thank him for publishing his books, and for clarification of the above.  I was not able to get through to him, or to Dr. Phyllis Balch.

There is some research that suggests Chromium Picolinate should be replaced with Chromium Polynicotinate because of safety concerns.  There is a report out that suggests the Picolinate version can actually affect our DNA.  A recent study found that chromium picolinate triggered potentially cancer-causing cell mutations in animals.  However, the chromium needed to affect humans in a similar way is a much larger amount than we could get from our supplements.  This questionable concern will take further research to confirm or deny the importance of the allegation.

In my on-going research, I have found several sources touting the benefit of folic acid for diabetics.  I now take this in 800 mcg tablets.  There is often the suggestion that folic acid be taken with B-12.  I take two of the 500 mcg's of the B-12 with folic acid.  Surprising, there is also a benefit for the heart.  Homocysteine has been identified as a principal cause of heart attacks.  It seems that high levels of this potent threat to a healthy heart can occur when protein is ineffectively converted in our bodies.  Folic acid and B-12 counterattack the homocysteine. It is suggested that we get homocysteine levels periodically checked.  For diabetics, it is great to know that as we reduce diabetes in our bodies, we are also protecting our hearts from this particular threat.

There is a new form of Folic Acid, Foliate, which is said to help the absorption of the Folic Acid. This too needs more research. It is an interesting area because in taking supplements, our body may not be absorbing all that we are paying for.

We discussed earlier, in the section Herbs and Other Recommendations, that flavonoids are good for the diabetic. I identified grape seed extract, and pine bark extract. I take 50 mg each now and then. The pine bark extract is known as Pycogenol. These two herbs are important to vascular health and circulation. This sounds good for neuropathy treatment or prevention. They may have an effect on those taking blood thinners, so you should discuss taking them with your doctor, and identify appropriate dosages.

Figure 4, on the next page, provide you with a modified listing of supplements. It is the version that helped me in my fight to rid myself of diabetes. You may want to copy it and put it on the back of your medicine cabinet door.

As you progress on your program, always vigilant to maintain the success of supplements and diet, and getting back on the program if you slip, you should also see yourself as unique. We are all somewhat different, and you <u>are</u> in charge of your own health.

You may want to experiment with some supplement dosages. You could reduce the dosage, say about a third, and evaluate the affect on your glucose reading. If the result consistently has little or no affect on your number, stay with the change because it could save you money. You should not stop a supplement because as we have learned, many times a supplement to fight diabetes is also helping your body in other ways.

## *Masison Modified Supplement List*

Group A      Essential

(2 a day)     L-Glutamine, Taurine, and L-Carnitine @500 mg    Alpha Lipoic @ 300 mg

(1 a day)     Chromium, Biotin @ 600 mcg     Zinc @ 50 mg     C-Q-10 @ 100 mg


Group B      Very Important

(1 a day)     Magnesium @ 500 mg     Manganese @ 10 mg

               Vitamin C @ 3000 mg     Vitamin E @ 1200 IU

               Beta Carotene @ 15 mg     Vitamin B-6 @ 100 mg


Group C      Important

(1 a day)     Selenium @ 200 mcg    Potassium @ 99 mg    Coral Calcium w/D @ 400 mg

               Bilberry @ 80 mg    Flax Seeds, Walnuts    Pycnogenol @ 50 mg

               Spirulina can be helpful for the hypoglycemia.  Recommend taking it between

               meals.


Group D    B-12 @ 1000 mcg    Folic Acid @ 800 mcg

              B-12 should be taken alone, or only with Folic Acid.

You may want to try fenugreek or gymnema and see if they help your program.


If for economical or other reasons, you will not be able to take all of the supplements, at least take the essential and very important.

If for any reason you miss taking some of the supplements one day, skip them.  Do not try to make up and take double the amount.


Figure 4

## *What About Multi-Vitamins?*

Usually the dosage, mcg's or mg's required to fight diabetes, are too large to be seen in a multi-vitamin. When you select a multi-vitamin to help maintain a healthy immune system, or use as part of a diabetic program, choose wisely says Dr. Jeffrey Blumberg, Professor of Nutrition at Tufts University.[7] He says choose a multi that is close to 100% of the Daily Value (DV) of most of the essential vitamins and minerals. Dr. Helen Delichhatsios of the Harvard Medical School[8] advice to us is to select one that has part or all of its Vitamin A as the safer beta-carotene.

As for slow-release multi's, Dr. Blumberg says there's not enough evidence that they offer any advantage to offset the extra cost. It may seem to many to take multi's that also contain herbs, but Dr. Blumberg says it's not a good idea. "Herbs are not nutrients; they are taken for very specific effects in the body."

It seems to me that using vitamins, herbs and minerals in the dosages that have been researched by qualified nutritional experts, to combat diseases, makes sense, as I have discovered in ridding myself of diabetes. I have written to two supplement makers, suggesting that they combine 2 or 3 supplements at the right dosages into a diabetic multi. For example, Taurine, Glutamine, and L-Carnitine, all at 500 mg. Care must be taken to not combine some supplements. An example would be calcium and manganese. Also, do not combine B-12 with any other supplement, other than folic acid.

Dr. Blumberg and Dr. Delichhatsios' comments are pertinent to the standard multi taken to enhance the immune system. They also provide some insights that are valuable to our basic

---

[7] Prevention Magazine, June 2003
[8] Prevention Magazine, June 2003

health and to diabetes. The hope here is that some research be undertaken to develop diabetic specific multis that can make taking them easier, and hopefully less expensive.

I also refer the reader back to the multi labeled <u>Doctor's Choice for Diabetes.</u> In this multi, there were 14 supplements. Four from the essential list, recommended by the Balch's were not in there. C-Q-10 from the very important list was not included. Dosages were minimal. Not one of the 14 supplements made the list, or they had less dosages needed to realistically fight diabetes in the program that I was following.

We all will look forward to a multi or two that will be a combination of supplements being used in the <u>Fight Diabetes Program</u>.

## The Silver Bullet Supplement

The "silver bullet" has been labeled in the history of medicine, as the one attack item that can be fired at a particular disease or ailment, to defeat (cure) it. It has a special allure because it simplifies things, tends to promise a quick cure, and it should be a fairly inexpensive treatment. There have been many such "silver bullets" suggested in the course of medical history.

Recently, a lady asked me if diabetes could be beaten by only taking magnesium. She had read that it could, and her friends were talking about it. I said that I doubted it. I said that magnesium definitely helps in the battle, but my experience is that it takes more than the magnesium, or any single supplement, to defeat diabetes. I explained to her that there were many recent claims of a single supplement "curing" diabetes. This included fenugreek, vinegar, cinnamon, spirulina, blueberries, and several others.

Some in the medical community find that one of our recommended supplements does a good job in one part of the diabetes fight, and jumps on it as a cure-all for diabetes. Carnitine and magnesium are examples.

I don't believe I would have achieved readings of 103 to 108 with only some of the supplements. I believe that a single supplement approach must also include the right diet, the source of the diabetes, to have any realistic value.

You know what is coming next. Take your reading for a week. Then stop the Fight Diabetes Program. Try the "magic potion" for a while, and see if you rid yourself of diabetes. Use your "test laboratory" to verify the claim for the silver bullet.

There are many in this world that would be delighted to come up with a single item solution, and a specific diet, say of pineapple. They really mean right but in using the self-test approach, you can stay grounded in the real world.

## *Eye Exam for Older Diabetics*

Diabetes is the leading cause of blindness in adults aged 20 to 74. More than 24,000 new cases of diabetes-related blindness are reported each year.

A major initiative aimed at reducing visual loss among diabetics is being co-sponsored by the American Academy of Ophthalmology and the American Optometric Association, along with the Federal Health Care Financing Administration.

If you're 65 or older, have diabetes, and have not had a medical eye exam in three years, call the National Eye Care Project Help line. It is 1-800-222-EYES and it is operating 24 hours per day.

They will put you in touch with an ophthalmologist who, at no cost to you, will provide you with an eye exam and up to a year of follow-up care for any condition diagnosed at that exam.

While you are undertaking what we can call a diabetic improvement program, it would not be prudent to pass up this opportunity to have a free eye exam, and free for any necessary follow-up.

## Reading List

This is a reading list, not quite the same as a reference list. I did not use all of the material listed here, in the book. I have included this non-referenced material, many of which I have only partially read, or not at all, in order to provide a fairly comprehensive information base for those wanting to thoroughly explore diabetes and their health in additional depth. The reader will decide whether to pursue them.

Prescription for Nutritional Healing (1997)
Dr. James Balch, Dr. Phyllis Balch
Avery Publishing Group
Garden City Park, New York

The Super Antioxidants (1998)
Dr. James Balch
M. Evans and Company, New York

The Glucose Revolution (1999)
Miller, Wolever, Colagiuri, Powell
Marlowe & Company, New York

New Diet Revolution (1992)
Dr. Robert Atkins
Avon Books, Harper Collins
New York, New York

The Hidden Causes of Most Illness (1998)
Dr. Atkins Health Revelations
Baltimore, MD

8 Weeks to Optimum Health (1997)
Andrew Weil, M.D.
Random House, Association w/Alfred A. Knopf, Inc.

Uncommon Cures for Everyday Ailments
Bottom Line Health
Boardroom Inc., 55 Railroad Ave.
Greenwich, CT 06830

Sugar Busters Shoppers' Guide (1999)
Steward, Bethea, Andrews, Balart
Ballantine Books, New York

Bottom Line Health
Bottom Line Books
PO Box 1400
Des Moines, IA 50381-1400

Minding the Body, Mending the Mind (1998)
Fire in the Soul (1988)
Joan Borysenko
Bantam Books, Addison-Wesley
Reading, MA

The Silva Mind Control Method (1977)
Jose Silva
Pocket Books, 1230 Avenue of the Americas
New York, NY 10020

Homeopathic Medicine (1995)
Ulman & Ulman
Picnic Point Press, Edward, WA

The Herbal Drugstore (2000)
Linda White, Steven Foster
Rodale, Inc.

Fit for Life I and II (1985, 1987)
Harvey and Marilyn Diamond
Warner Books, New York, NY

Rid Yourself of Diabetes (1999)
Charles J. Masison
1st Books, Bloomington, IN

Healing Words (1993)
Larry Dossey, MD
Harper Collins, San Francisco

Healing Beyond the Body (2001)
Larry Dossey, MD
Shambhala
Boston and London

Anatomy of an Illness (1979)
Norman Cousins
Bantam

Ageless Body, Timeless Mind (1993)
Depak Chopra
Crown Publications

How to Stop Worrying (1975)
Dale Carnegie
Simon & Schuster

Stop Aging Now (1996)
Jean Carper
HarperCollins Publisher
New York

Advanced Nutritional Therapies (1982)
Dr. Kenneth Cooper
Thomas Nelson Publishing, Nashville

Protein Power (1996)
Dr. Michael Eades, Dr. Mary Dan Eades
Bantam Books, New York

The Zone (1995)
Barry Sears, Bill Lawren
Regan Books, New York

The South Beach Diet (2003)
Arthur Agatston, MD
Rodale Inc,

Health & Nutrition Letter (2004)
Weighing In On the South Beach Diet
Tufts University
The Friedman Guide to Living Healthier Longer

Creative Visualization (1978)
Shakti Gawain
Whatever Publishing Inc.
San Rafael, CA

How You Can Use The Technique of Creative Imagination (1988)
Roy Eugene Davis
CSA Press, Publishers
Lakemont, GA

Doctor, What Should I Eat (1995)
Isadore Rosenfeld, MD
Random House
New York

Magazine – Diabetes Interview (03-04)
Fairfax, CA

Alternatives (Spring 2004)
Mountain Home Publishing
PO Box 61010
Rockville, MD 20859-1010
(Issue Volume 9, No 26)

Live Right for Your Type (2001)
Dr. Peter J. D'Adamo
G.P. Putnam's Sons
New York, NY

*Winning The Fight Against Diabetes Order Form*


Send me copies of *Winning the Fight Against Diabetes* for me and my friends

_____copies at $14.95 a copy for paperback        Total $_____

_____copies at $24.95 a copy for hardcover        Total $_____


You can trade in a copy of *Rid Yourself of Diabetes* for a discount of $5.00 towards

the purchase of *Winning The Fight Against Diabetes,* by forwarding the front cover.


Tomorrows Health Today Publishers
PO Box 113
Foxboro, MA 02035

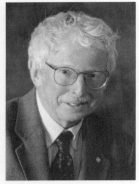

Charles Masison has been an active explorer of traditional and alternative health practices. He has developed a strong capability in nutritional healing, with a concentration in diabetes.

In analyzing nutritional research from around the world, he has integrated several healing approaches into a proven program. The results of this research have proven beneficial to many in ridding their bodies of diabetes.

Masison demonstrated which of the healing techniques really works, by testing them on his own body. He was able to bring his diabetic glucose reading of 168 down to a non-diabetic 103. This is well below the American Diabetes Association standard for a non-diabetic of 120. Masison believes adult-onset diabetics can follow the program that he developed, and that they can achieve similar results.

With the diabetic epidemic now rapidly spreading to 40 and 50 year olds, the increase in American diabetics is now estimated at greater than a million per year. This book becomes compelling reading for the adult-onset diabetic and for those who wish to avoid getting the disease.

Masison first identified the usefulness of the Atkins diet in 1999. He supported the assertion that the medical community's claim that a low fat diet was necessary for good health as a myth. Using his own body, he developed clinical proof to show that the low fat diet was not a serious threat to one's health.

Masison has gone beyond traditional thinking and identified millions of Americans who are diabetic but not being treated to fight this silent killer. He advocates physicians evaluate his premises, and incorporate his thoughts on diagnosing the disease based on a deviation from their glucose standard rather than acceptance of a value within a range. The physician's patients may need the treatment and care of a diabetic before they are faced with neuropathy, macular degeneration, and other serious complications of diabetes.

Masison's program is based on reviewing many sources of nutritional research. This research has now been analyzed by this MIT graduate, using the scientific method familiar to researchers and physicians in the medical community. The results of his analysis have been made useful to those fighting diabetes.

The 60-day, self-help program, is the start of winning the fight against diabetes.